Telehealth in Otolaryngology

Guest Editors

MICHAEL R. HOLTEL, MD
YEHUDAH ROTH, MD

OTOLARYNGOLOGIC CLINICS OF NORTH AMERICA

www.oto.theclinics.com

December 2011 • Volume 44 • Number 6

SAUNDERS an imprint of ELSEVIER, Inc.

W.B. SAUNDERS COMPANY
A Division of Elsevier Inc.

1600 John F. Kennedy Boulevard • Suite 1800 • Philadelphia, Pennsylvania 19103-2899

http://www.theclinics.com

OTOLARYNGOLOGIC CLINICS OF NORTH AMERICA Volume 44, Number 6
December 2011 ISSN 0030-6665, ISBN-13: 978-1-4557-1114-7

Editor: Joanne Husovski
Developmental Editor: Donald Mumford

Otolaryngologic Clinics of North America (ISSN 0030-6665) is published bimonthly by Elsevier, Inc., 360 Park Avenue South, New York, NY 10010-1710. Months of issue are February, April, June, August, October, and December. Business and Editorial Offices: 1600 John F. Kennedy Blvd., Suite 1800, Philadelphia, PA 19103-2899. Customer Service Office: 6277 Sea Harbor Drive, Orlando, FL 32887-4800. Periodicals postage paid at New York, NY and additional mailing offices. Subscription prices is $310.00 per year (US individuals), $590.00 per year (US institutions), $149.00 per year (US student/resident), $409.00 per year (Canadian individuals), $741.00 per year (Canadian institutions), $459.00 per year (international individuals), $741.00 per year (international institutions), $230.00 per year (international & Canadian student/resident). Foreign air speed delivery is included in all *Clinics'* subscription prices. All prices are subject to change without notice. **POSTMASTER:** Send address changes to *Otolaryngologic Clinics of North America*, Elsevier Health Sciences Division, Subscription Customer Service, 3251 Riverport Lane, Maryland Heights, MO 63043. **Telephone: 1-800-654-2452 (U.S. and Canada); 314-447-8871 (outside U.S. and Canada). Fax: 314-447-8029. E-mail: journalscustomerservice-usa@elsevier.com (for print support); journalsonlinesupport-usa@elsevier.com (for online support).**

Reprints. For copies of 100 or more of articles in this publication, please contact the Commercial Reprints Department, Elsevier Inc., 360 Park Avenue South, New York, NY 10010-1710. Tel.: 212-633-3812; Fax: 212-462-1935; E-mail: reprints@elsevier.com.

Otolaryngologic Clinics of North America is also published in Spanish by McGraw-Hill Interamericana Editores S.A., P.O. Box 5-237, 06500 Mexico D.F., Mexico.

Otolaryngologic Clinics of North America is covered in *MEDLINE/PubMed (Index Medicus), Current Contents/Clinical Medicine, Excerpta Medica, BIOSIS, Science Citation Index,* and *ISI/BIOMED.*

Printed and bound by CPI Group (UK) Ltd, Croydon, CR0 4YY

Transferred to Digital Print 2011

Contributors

GUEST EDITORS

MICHAEL R. HOLTEL, MD, FACS
Sharp Rees-Stealy Medical Group, San Diego; Associate Professor, University of Hawaii; Senior Advisor, Acoustic Trauma, Telemedicine, and Advanced Technology Research Center Fort Detrick, Maryland

YEHUDAH ROTH, MD
Canada International Scientific Exchange Program; Department of Public Health Sciences, University of Toronto, Toronto, Canada; Edith Wolfson Medical Center, Tel Aviv University Sackler School of Medicine, Holon, Israel; The Peter A. Silverman Centre for International Health, Mount Sinai Hospital, Toronto, Canada

AUTHORS

ZIAD ABDEEN, PhD
Canada International Scientific Exchange Program, Toronto, Canada; Al Quds University, Abu Dis, West Bank; Department of Public Health Sciences, University of Toronto, Toronto, Canada

MOISÉS ARRIAGA, MD, MBA, FACS
Clinical Professor of Otolaryngology and Neurosurgery, Director of Otology/Neurotology, LSU Health Science Center, New Orleans, Louisiana; Medical Director, Hearing and Balance Center, Our Lady of the Lake Regional Medical Center, Baton Rouge, Louisiana

REBECCA Y. ARRIAGA, M Litt
Operations Director 1, Our Lady of the Lake Physicians Group, Our Lady of the Lake Regional Medical Center, Baton Rouge, Louisiana

SANDRA BLACK, MD, FRCPC
Division of Neurology, Department of Medicine, Sunnybrook Health Sciences Centre, Rotman Research Institute, University of Toronto, Toronto, Canada

JANET E. BROWN, MA
Director, Health Care Services in Speech-Language Pathology, American Speech-Language-Hearing Association, Rockville, Maryland

ZIAD ELNASSER, MD, PhD
Canada International Scientific Exchange Program; Department of Public Health Sciences, University of Toronto, Toronto, Canada; King Abdulla University Hospital, Jordan University of Science and Technology, Irbid, Jordan

A. STEWART FERGUSON, PhD
Alaska Native Tribal Health Consortium, Anchorage, Alaska

MORRIS FREEDMAN, MD, FRCPC
Division of Neurology, Department of Medicine, Mt Sinai Hospital, Rotman Research Institute, Baycrest, University and Health Network, University of Toronto, Toronto, Canada

FRANK G. GARRITANO, MD
Division of Otolaryngology–Head and Neck Surgery, Department of Surgery, Penn State Hershey Medical Center, Hershey, Pennsylvania

DAVID GOLDENBERG, MD, FACS
Division of Otolaryngology–Head and Neck Surgery, Department of Surgery, Penn State Hershey Medical Center, Hershey, Pennsylvania

KELLY L. GROOM, MD
Division of Otolaryngology, Tripler Army Medical Center, Honolulu, Hawaii

MICHAEL R. HOLTEL, MD, FACS
Sharp Rees-Stealy Medical Group, San Diego; Associate Professor, University of Hawaii; Senior Advisor, Acoustic Trauma, Telemedicine, and Advanced Technology Research Center Fort Detrick, Maryland

ANDREW IGNATIEFF, BA
Canada International Scientific Exchange Program; The Peter A. Silverman Centre for International Health, Mount Sinai Hospital, Toronto, Canada

JESSICA I. KENYON, MA
Director of Operations, US Army Telemedicine and Advanced Technology Research Center (TATRC), West Coast Satellite Office, US Army Medical Research and Materiel Command (USAMRMC), Marina del Rey, California

JOHN KOKESH, MD
Alaska Native Medical Center, Anchorage, Alaska

MARK KRUMM, PhD
Associate Professor in Audiology, North East Ohio AuD Consortium (NOAC); Department of Speech Pathology and Audiology, Kent State University, Kent, Ohio

ELIZABETH A. KRUPINSKI, PhD
Professor and Vice Chair of Radiology, Department of Radiology, University of Arizona, Tucson, Arizona

RONALD B. KUPPERSMITH, MD, MBA, FACS
Clinical faculty, Texas A&M Health Science Center, College Station, Texas

PAULINE A. MASHIMA, PhD
Chief, Otolaryngology Service, Speech Pathology Section, Tripler Army Medical Center; Adjunct Graduate Faculty, Department of Communication Sciences and Disorders, University of Hawaii, Honolulu, Hawaii

JASON G. NEWMAN, MD, FACS
Assistant Professor, Department of Otorhinolaryngology–Head and Neck Surgery, The University of Pennsylvania Health System, Philadelphia, Pennsylvania

CAMERON D. NORMAN, PhD
Director of Evaluation, Peter A. Silverman Global eHealth Program, Dalla Lana School of Public Health; Canada International Scientific Exchange Program; Department of Public Health Sciences, University of Toronto, Toronto, Ontario, Canada

ARNOLD NOYEK, MD, FRCSC
Canada International Scientific Exchange Program, Toronto, Canada; Al Quds University, Abu Dis, West Bank; Department of Public Health Sciences, University of Toronto, Toronto, Canada; The Peter A. Silverman Centre for International Health, Mount Sinai Hospital; Department of Otolaryngology–Head and Neck Surgery, University of Toronto; Director, International Continuing Education, University of Toronto, Faculty of Medicine, Toronto, Canada

DANIEL NUSS, MD, FACS
Professor and Chairman, LSU Department of Otorhinolaryngology Head and Neck Surgery, New Orleans, Louisiana

BERT W. O'MALLEY Jr, MD
Gabriel Tucker Professor, Department of Otorhinolaryngology–Head and Neck Surgery, The University of Pennsylvania Health System, Philadelphia, Pennsylvania

CHRIS PATRICOSKI, MD
Alaska Native Tribal Health Consortium, Anchorage, Alaska

TIM PATTERSON, BA
Telehealth Coordinator, Baycrest; Canada International Scientific Exchange Program, Toronto, Canada; Al Quds University, Abu Dis, West Bank

COLONEL RONALD POROPATICH, MD
Deputy Director, US Army Telemedicine and Advanced Technology Research Center (TATRC), US Army Medical Research and Materiel Command (USAMRMC), Fort Detrick, Maryland

MITCHELL J. RAMSEY, MD
Division of Otolaryngology, Tripler Army Medical Center, Honolulu, Hawaii

YEHUDAH ROTH, MD
Canada International Scientific Exchange Program; Department of Public Health Sciences, University of Toronto, Toronto, Canada; Edith Wolfson Medical Center, Tel Aviv University Sackler School of Medicine, Holon, Israel; The Peter A. Silverman Centre for International Health, Mount Sinai Hospital, Toronto, Canada

JAMES E. SAUNDERS, MD
Department of Otolaryngology, Dartmouth Medical Center, Lebanon, New Hampshire

GIL SIEGAL, MD (TAU), LLB (TAU), SJD (UVa)
Professor of Law, University of Virginia School of Law, Charlottesville, Virginia; Senior Surgeon, Department of Otolaryngology–Head and Neck Surgery, Tel Hashomer Hospital; Director, Center for Health Law, Bioethics and Health Policy, Kiryat Ono College, Israel

ABI SRIHARAN, MSc
The Peter A. Silverman Centre for International Health, Mount Sinai Hospital, Toronto, Canada

DON STREDNEY, MA
Departments of Otolaryngology and Biomedical Informatics, Ohio Supercomputer Center, The Ohio State University, Columbus, Ohio

MARK J. SYMS, MD, FACS
Neurotology, Barrow Neurological Institute; Director, Arizona Ear Center, Phoenix, Arizona

DINAH WAN, MD
College of Medicine, The Ohio State University, Columbus, Ohio

GREGORY J. WIET, MD, FACS, FAAP
Departments of Otolaryngology and Biomedical Informatics, The Ohio State University, Columbus, Ohio

Contents

> The opportunity to treat neurotologic patients when the patient and physician are in separate locations is an important clinical delivery mechanism. The authors developed their applications of neurotologic telemedicine in the aftermath of Hurricane Katrina and found this to be an effective way to deliver clinical care, develop a clinical neurotology practice, and train residents and fellows and to manage a growing neurotologic clinical practice remotely. This article outlines the technical requirements, current uses, clinical applicability, and implementation details of the Our Lady of the Lake – LSU neurotology telemedicine program; administrative issues surrounding telemedicine; and future considerations.

> A significant worldwide need exists for humanitarian assistance in the specialty of otolaryngology. The field of telehealth has provided applications that have successfully expanded access to care in many fields of medicine, in both developed and developing countries. Collaboration, planning, and persistence are essential to developing successful telehealth applications. This article describes the need for otolaryngologic specialty care, current humanitarian outreach within the field of otolaryngology, and examples of successful programs that incorporate telehealth in otolaryngology care.

> This article discusses the types of telemedicine technologies that are currently in place and being used successfully in otolaryngology. It examines how these technologies have been applied in several different otolaryngology telemedicine programs and discusses their relative merits and successes.

> Telemedicine and telehealth programs are generally more complex than their traditional on-site health care delivery counterparts. A few organizations have developed sustainable, multispecialty telemedicine programs, but single service programs, such as teleradiology and teledermatology, are common. Planning and maintaining a successful telemedicine program

is challenging, and there are often barriers to developing sustainable telehealth programs. This article reviews some important aspects of developing a telehealth program, and provides two examples of currently operating successful model programs.

discussion includes an overview of key topics in training and learning, the application of these issues in simulation environments, and the subsequent applications of these simulation environments to otolaryngology. Examples of past applications are presented, with discussion of how the interplay of cultural changes in surgical training in general along with the rapid advancements in technology have shaped and influenced their adoption and adaptation. The authors conclude with emerging trends and potential influences advanced simulation and training will have on technical skills training in otolaryngology.

FORTHCOMING ISSUES

Cochlear Implants
J. Thomas Roland, MD, and
David Haynes, MD, *Guest Editors*

Vestibular Schwannoma
Fred Telischi, MD, and
Jacques Morcos, MD,
Guest Editors

**Pediatric Otolaryngology Challenges
in Multi-System Disease**
Austin Rose, MD, *Guest Editor*

RECENT ISSUES

Neurorhinology: Complex Lesions
Richard J. Harvey, MD, and
Carl H. Snyderman, MD, *Guest Editors*
October 2011

Neurorhinology: Common Pathologies
Richard J. Harvey, MD, and
Carl Snyderman, MD, *Guest Editors*
August 2011

Allergies for the Otolaryngologist
B.J. Ferguson, MD, and
Suman Golla, MD, *Guest Editors*
June 2011

RELATED INTEREST

American Journal of Preventive Medicine, May 2011 (Volume 40, Issue 5,
Supplement 2) Pages S162–S172
Promise of and Potential for Patient-Facing Technologies to Enable Meaningful Use
David K. Ahern, Susan S. Woods, Marie C. Lightowler, Scott W. Finley, and
Thomas K. Houston

THE CLINICS ARE NOW AVAILABLE ONLINE!

Access your subscription at:
www.theclinics.com

Preface

A Toy Story?

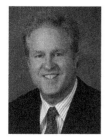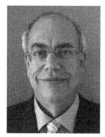

Michael R. Holtel, MD   Yehudah Roth, MD
Guest Editors

While advocates see Telehealth as an essential fundamental change that will improve the way health care is delivered, others view Telehealth as a nice-to-have-tool or an intriguing array of high-tech gadgets, which may make us feel "cutting edge" but ultimately have little effect on the delivery of care. Some of its harshest critics see it as an expensive and time-consuming operation that is unlikely to enhance the existing health care system.

While not a challenge for the average adolescent, there are clearly challenges in the transition to new or different communication modalities in the adult population. While we all watch television and often enjoy the various interactive programs as passive observers, when a group of professionals convene and are asked to communicate with a similar remote group using analogous television techniques, an interesting spectrum of avoidance and hesitant attitudes appears that frequently hinders successful encounter, regardless if it is a Continuing Medical Education event, active consultation, or telesurgery.

More passive, less interactive applications, such as electronic medical records, are understandably more acceptable, although we all share the frustrations, sometimes anger, that exist around their implementation and inefficiencies. Our profession is many times a solo venture encompassing long hours, either in the clinic or in the operating room. Unidirectional encounters, such as patient education or even e-prescriptions, are often more intuitively comfortable, while electronic interactive exchange tends to meet with more resistance, often reflected as skepticism.

PUTTING COMMUNICATIONS IN ORDER

To firm believers, such as the editors, the use of a computer or mobile devices, camera, software, and good communication lines seems natural. The enormous improvements that telemedicine can bring about to our profession, the provision of

Otolaryngol Clin N Am 44 (2011) xi–xiii
doi:10.1016/j.otc.2011.09.003
0030-6665/11/$ – see front matter © 2011 Elsevier Inc. All rights reserved.

better care to large populations, the higher standards of care, and the advancement of technology are promising. With the rapid advent of access to the Internet, increasing Internet speed (Internet 2.0), and increasing use of mini-computers, smart phones, and mobile devices, we will witness in the forthcoming years increasingly useful applications. Hopefully, we will also see improved and wise management strategies as well as user-friendly administrative and regulatory approaches.

It is becoming apparent that the worldwide cost of mobile devices and communication has reached a level that makes these commodities widely available and affordable. In parallel, interest of consumers increases exponentially, although it is focused among younger people. Like many new technologies, adoption by the older generation follows.

eHealth is becoming a strong and rapidly evolving industry. Several fields are emerging within this trade. Mobile health monitoring is a broad category, involving now-termed traditional issues such as glucose and blood pressure monitoring, and newer biometric remote monitoring solutions via wearable devices or smart phones that may monitor health and fitness habits, balance, voice, hearing, rehabilitation exercises, or adherence to medications.

Interactive real-time telemedicine services, as one form of telemedicine, include phone or video conversations, up to virtual home visits, which may provide history review, some measure of physical examination, and mental and behavioral evaluations, which are comparable to those done in traditional encounters. These services may be less costly than in-person clinical visits.

Some diagnostic medical devices may be mobilized and used in underserviced areas. Tele-audiology and tele-neurootology are good examples. Remote robotics is currently limited in testing and implementation, due to the high cost of development, integration, stretched operation, and maintenance learning curves. We share the belief that this will develop in our field as well and will enable the deployment of sophisticated surgical services in more detached places. The importance of mobilizing services is strongly demonstrated in various disaster scenario and humanitarian ventures.

Short Message Service SMS-based appointment reminders and prescription reminders, specific notification of completed lab results, in addition to basic fitness and wellness applications, are becoming prevalent, improve administrative efficiency, and, with the evolution of social health-care-oriented communities, render more responsibility of personal wellness to the patients rather than solely relying on health care professionals. These are reflections of a fascinating on-going social and psychological transformation.

The privacy and security concerns associated with the electronic transmission of health care information are an important consideration. The Health Insurance Portability and Accountability Act, the Health Information Technology for Economic and Clinical Health Act, and their surrounding regulations and guidelines demonstrate the difficulties and attempted solutions to integrate eHealth applications into evolving social changes.

GOAL

The intent of this issue is to present to the readership an updated overview of the field, to point out the fascinating challenges, and to encourage our colleagues to see the potential of this rapidly growing industry.

THANK YOU

We are grateful for the authors herein who share with us their experiences, lessons, and critical reflections, and to Joanne Husovski, Senior Editor at Elsevier, for her ongoing encouragement, patience, and efficiency, which enabled this transoceanic project.

Michael R. Holtel, MD
Otolaryngology–Head and Neck Surgery
Sharp Rees Stealy
10670 Wexford Street
San Diego, CA 92131, USA

Telemedicine Research Institute
John A. Burns School of Medicine
University of Hawaii
651 Ilalo Street
Honolulu, HI 96813, USA

Telemedicine and Advanced Technology Research Center of the United States
States Army Medical Readiness and Materiel Command
Building, 1054 Patchel Street
Fort Detrick, MD 21702, USA

Yehudah Roth, MD
Department of Otolaryngology–Head and Neck Surgery
Edith Wolfson Medical Center
Tel Aviv University Sackler Faculty of Medicine
62 HaLohamim Street, PO Box 5
Holon 58100, Israel

E-mail addresses:
mholtel@hawaii.edu (M.R. Holtel)
orl@wolfson.helath.gov.il (Y. Roth)

Neurotology Telemedicine Consultation

Moisés Arriaga, MD, MBA[a,b,*], Daniel Nuss, MD[c],
Rebecca Y. Arriaga, M Litt[d]

KEYWORDS

- Neurotology • Telemedicine • Natural disaster
- Health care delivery

Key Points: NEUROTOLOGY TELECONSULTATION

- Neurotology is well suited for delivery through telemedicine, and this delivery method is particularly useful in underserved areas or in times of natural disaster.
- Basic technical requirements for neurotologic telemedicine are a codec, video otoscopy, infrared video eye movement recording, an otoscopist at the patient end, digital access to imaging, technical support at the patient and provider locations, and secure data transmission.
- Legal requirements usually include medical licensure at the patient and provider locations.
- Reimbursement is location-specific, with clear guidelines in rural areas. Reimbursement in other areas requires specific discussions with insurers and government programs.

The opportunity to treat neurotologic patients when the patient and physician are in separate locations is an important clinical delivery mechanism. The authors developed their applications of neurotologic telemedicine in the aftermath of Hurricane Katrina and found this to be an effective way to deliver clinical care, develop a clinical neurotology practice, and train residents and fellows and to manage a growing neurotologic

---

[a] Lousiana State University Health Science Center, New Orleans, LA, USA
[b] Hearing and Balance Center Our Lady of the Lake Regional Medical Center, 7777 Hennessey Boulevard, Suite 709, Baton Rouge, LA 70808, USA
[c] Lousiana State University Department of Otorhinolaryngology Head and Neck Surgery, 533 Bolivar Street, New Orleans, LA 70112, USA
[d] Our Lady of the Lake Physicians Group, Our Lady of the Lake Regional Medical Center, 7777 Hennessy Boulevard, Baton Rouge, LA 70808, USA
* Corresponding author.
E-mail address: maa@neurotologic.com

Otolaryngol Clin N Am 44 (2011) 1235–1250
doi:10.1016/j.otc.2011.08.001
0030-6665/11/$ – see front matter © 2011 Elsevier Inc. All rights reserved.

clinical practice remotely. This article outlines the technical requirements, current uses, clinical applicability, and implementation details of the Our Lady of the Lake – Louisiana State University (LSU) neurotology telemedicine program; administrative issues surrounding telemedicine; and future considerations. Although the initial program was a necessary step to maintain clinical services and the otolaryngology residency after Hurricane Katrina, the benefits have extended far beyond the initial intent, including identifying a practical technique to extend services to underserved areas and potentially help alleviate the pending shortage of otolaryngologists.

Telemedicine is a mode of health care delivery in which the physician is able to care for a patient when the patient and physician are not in the same place at the same time. Like other applications of telemedicine, neurotology applications of telemedicine can occur as real-time encounters or as delayed (store-and-forward) interactions. Because neurotology relies heavily on visualization of the ear, imaging studies, physiologic evaluations of balance, and review of electrophysiologic studies, the technical requirements lend themselves to widespread application of telemedicine.

The use of telemedicine as a delivery tool for otology and neurotology has grown beyond a novel theoretical consideration, because telemedicine is now a practical and viable clinical delivery method. This article reviews several aspects, presented in **Box 1**.

TECHNICAL REQUIREMENTS AND OPTIONS FOR NEUROTOLOGY TELEMEDICINE

For store-and-forward neurotology telemedicine, any system that allows recording of images and or videos for later viewing, interpretation, and treatment recommendations is applicable. These types of efforts have been particularly useful in rural outreach where many patients' ears are examined and recorded by an advance screening team with later transmission of the data to experts at a central location.[1] Furthermore, these systems have been validated and compared with on-site otoscopy documenting the accuracy of the technique for otologic diagnosis.[2] High-quality otoendoscopes and computer software with the ability to record and transmit digital images permit accurate visualization of ear canal and tympanic membrane pathology.

For real-time telemedicine, the needs are more complex. A codec unit is the centerpiece. This unit permits teleconferencing, including not only traditional video and audio but also the ability to connect additional input sources, such as the video endoscope for otoendoscopy, digital stethoscope, fiber optic laryngeal endoscopy, infrared video camera for eye movement recording, and digital transmission of overhead projections of imaging films/paper documents, and real-time computer display of word processing and slide presentation software. Tandberg and Polycom manufacture units with easy compatibility. **Figs. 1** and **2** show two of the codec units used by the authors. Price for these devices and peripheral configurations ranges from approximately $10,000 to several hundred thousand dollars for multisite configurations. Factors influencing selection include screen size, space availability, technical expertise available for customization, and the compatibility of the peripheral devices selected.

Beyond the basic equipment, software configuration and negotiating firewalls appropriately are necessary steps to initiate and maintain the functionality of the system. Clinicians planning a real-time telemedicine clinical program must specifically consider the availability of information system resources to troubleshoot and expand the system, because Internet access, security issues, and program updates create a fluid situation requiring multisystem functionality.

Health Insurance Privacy and Portability Act (HIPPA) requirements are specific in the need for confidentiality. Security requirements are a necessary component of the system to maintain patient confidentiality. A VPN is one technique this program has

---

Box 1
Overview of neurotology telemedicine aspects

- Technical requirements and options for telemedicine
  - Codec
  - Content
  - Peripherals
  - Connectivity
  - Virtual private network (VPN)
- Current applications of otology and neurotology telemedicine
  - Otoscopy
  - Conferencing
  - Vestibular evaluation
  - Education
  - The diffusion of telemedicine in the United States and internationally
- Clinical applicability of neurotology telemedicine
  - Symptoms
  - Manpower considerations
  - Rural
  - Disaster
  - Training
  - Cochlear implant testing and programming
- Our Lady of the Lake – LSU Neurotology Telemedicine
  - Program organization
  - Patient satisfaction
  - Outcomes
- Administrative issues surrounding telemedicine
  - Consent
  - Malpractice insurance
  - Licensure
- Future consideration

---

found effective in creating a secure environment for patient communication. Using special username and password access, clinicians near and far can communicate freely about the patient, with access to the session permitted only to personnel with appropriate security access to the codes.

Peripheral inputs include the video endoscope tools described in the store-and-forward section. Endoscopic views of the ear canal and tympanic membrane can be taken real-time to adjust the view or focus on different aspects of the tympanic membrane or mastoid cavity. Additionally, magnified views can be obtained through connecting the office microscope to the codec, thus permitting otomicroscopy as a telemedicine tool. Facial function can be visualized with the high-resolution, remote

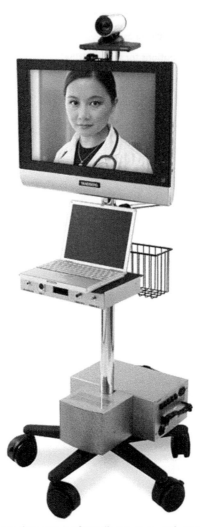

Fig. 1. Tandberg codec unit. (*Courtesy of* Tandberg, Inc.; with permission.)

zoom function of the video conferencing portion of the codec. Nystagmus evaluation is facilitated by infrared goggles and cameras, which permit nonfixation analysis of nystagmus and eye motion recording for positional, spontaneous, and gaze nystagmus. **Fig. 3** illustrates use of the Micromedical infrared goggles (Micromedical Technologies, Inc., Chatham, Illinois) during an actual telemedicine session with the author (MA) in Pittsburgh, Pennsylvania while the patient and neurotology fellow were in Baton Rouge, Louisiana during a Hallpike test for positional nystagmus.

The teleconferencing capabilities of the system require that the physician have control of camera position and zoom image of the patient's location. Similarly, both the patient and physician location need split-screen capabilities so that they can see an inset screen of their image being transmitted to the other party, and see each other. For neurotology, it is particularly useful for the physician to be able to manage multiple screen windows. In addition to visualizing the patient and himself,

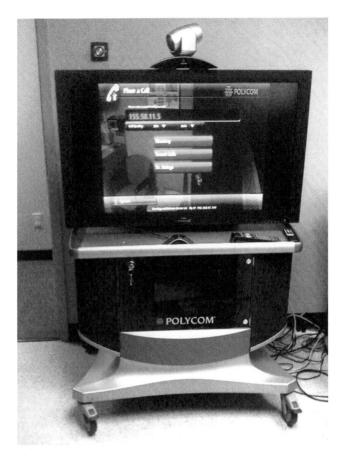

Fig. 2. Polycom telemedicine codec unit. (*Courtesy of* Moisés Arriaga, MD; with permission.)

the physician needs visualization of peripheral inputs, such as the video endoscope and infrared video goggles. For instance, during the Hallpike test, the physician can see the patient being placed in the Hallpike position while watching the infrared video camera transmission of their eye movements.

Additional content transmission during neurotology telemedicine sessions is also helpful for communication. In communicating with deaf and hard-of-hearing patients, one of the authors (MA) will switch to a word processing program using a large font display to close caption the conversation with the hard-of-hearing patient. In this manner, the communication is enhanced and both parties are sure the correct message has been relayed. Similarly, for patient education purposes during on-site patient encounters in neurotology, patient information pamphlets and brochures are often used to show normal and diseased physiology. With the telemedicine unit, physicians are able to switch to a slide presentation program during the visit to efficiently educate patients and their family during the patient visit.

CURRENT APPLICATIONS OF OTOLOGY AND NEUROTOLOGY TELEMEDICINE

Otoscopy is the most frequent current application of telemedicine in otology and neurotology. During outreach trips to underserved areas, recorded otoendoscope images

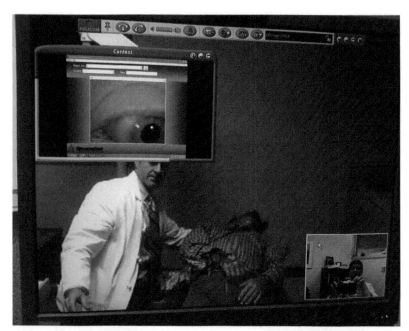

Fig. 3. Neurotology telemedicine in progress. This image was taken during a telemedicine session showing the patient in Baton Rouge, Louisiana with the assisting physician (neurotology fellow) placing the patient into the Hallpike position. The inset shows the infrared video eye images of the patient's eye movements visible to the assisting physician in Baton Rouge and the neurotologist (MA) in Pittsburgh, Pennsylvania. The bottom right inset shows the neurotologist in Pittsburgh taking this photograph of the screen during the telemedicine session. All the images on this photograph were visible in Pittsburgh and Baton Rouge during the telemedicine session. (*Courtesy of* Moisés Arriaga, MD; with permission.)

are transmitted to a central area with more specialized personnel than are available in the remote screening location. The Alaskan Telemedicine Project incorporates otoendoscopy as part of a complex telemedicine unit that is housed in various secondary centers closer to the patients' rural homes, which in turn transmits the images to a central location where more trained physicians and specialists can review the images and make recommendations.[3]

Special considerations in real-time neurotologic applications of otoendoscopy include ear canal moisture and focused views of different aspects of the tympanic membrane, ear canal, and mastoid cavity. A perforation with moisture can interfere with visualization of the tympanic membrane through fogging the lens. Generous application of antifog material, air puffs, and efficient placement and photography of the pathology can circumvent this limitation. The personnel maneuvering the endoscope need specific training and practice for accurate endoscopy. Particular skill is needed to understand what portion of the anatomy is necessary for visualizing pathology.

Teleconferencing can be considered the core capability of the codec unit, with visualization of peripheral inputs as add-on features. This core capability lends itself to applicant interviews and team conferences, even though the physician is not physically at the same office as the rest of the team.

The vestibular evaluation during a telemedicine session is similar to an on-site examination. The history is taken in a standard fashion using the teleconferencing function. The neurologic examination can include detailed cranial nerve examination, and endoscopic oral, pharyngeal, nasal, and even laryngeal examination. The camera can follow the patient in the examination room during gait, Romberg, and Fukuda step testing. Infrared goggles can evaluate for gaze and positional nystagmus, and even evaluate for fistula, Tullio phenomenon, hyperventilation, and vibration-induced nystagmus.

Similarly, telemedicine evaluations of patients with skull base lesions use the discussed functionalities. However, the patient education components are especially useful in skull base tumor and acoustic neuroma evaluations. Families particularly appreciate the real-time review of images showing the pathology, reviewing the anatomy, and discussing the treatment options. The conversation can be enhanced with brief PowerPoint presentations of computer slides.

Objective tinnitus is a specific symptom that requires auscultation in various head and neck sites for appropriate diagnosis. The digital stethoscope permits recording and transmission of sounds for diagnosis. This tool has been validated by its role in cardiology and remote physician evaluation/management of patients in intensive care units at distant locations.

Multiple Site Education

Resident, medical student, and ancillary staff education is facilitated by the teleconferencing capabilities. Since March 2006, the LSU Otolaryngology Department has had a regular telemedicine weekly lecture series highlighting simultaneous participation by faculty in numerous local, national, and international locations. Current participants in the lecture series include sites at Children's Hospital, New Orleans, LSU School of Allied Health, Our Lady of the Lake Regional Medical Center, Ohio Osteopathic Residency, Allegheny General Hospital, and Siglo 21 Medical Center in Mexico City. Because the teleconferencing functions use visualization and participation at the sites receiving and transmitting the lectures, the sessions can be truly interactive, with participants asking the presenter questions and the presenter able to quiz the participants on hypothetical cases and their mastery of the assigned reading material.

Diffusion of Telemedicine

Neurotology telemedicine is obviously a small part of telemedicine in modern medicine.[4] Accordingly, taking a step back to understand the process of incorporating this new innovation is important to understand the future role of telemedicine in neurotology.

In the mid 20th century, Everett Rogers[5] championed diffusion of innovation theory, which is still used to study the manner that new ideas spread. Diffusion, as explained by Rogers is, "the process by which an innovation is communicated through certain channels over time among members of social systems." Rogers defines an innovation as, "an idea, practice, or object perceived as new by an individual or other unit of adoption."[5] Rogers emphasizes that regardless of whether the adoption decision is planned, both uncertainty and the potential to create a social change are underlying characteristics of an innovation. The adoption of an innovation is a five-step process, which Rogers described as (1) learning about the innovation, (2) developing an attitude or opinion regarding the innovation, (3) deciding to accept or reject the innovation, (4) beginning to execute it, and (5) confirming the decision. The final step refers to the pivotal decisions adopters must make to integrate the innovation into their regular activities.[5]

A review of the five steps of the innovation adoption process shows that in the United States. telemedicine has surpassed the first stage of the process, learning about the innovation. This step represents gathering "how" and "why" knowledge about telemedicine. A simple search engine query for the terms "telemedicine" and "telehealth" shows a high volume of corresponding Web sites (**Fig. 4**). For example, a search for the term "telemedicine" at yahoo.com returned more than 9,000,000 results.[4]

Anecdotally, the idea of telemedicine has permeated the mainstream media, as evidenced by the new Cisco television commercial with Ellen Page. The commercial highlights the capabilities created by the use of telemedicine in a doctor's office. In the commercial, Page's doctor is on vacation in Copenhagen, yet he is still able to connect with the office and see patients.[6]

The second and third stages of the innovation adoption process are inextricably linked. The second stage focuses on the formation of an opinion about telemedicine, whereas the third stage emphasizes the decision to accept or reject telemedicine, a decision highly dependent on the opinion formed.[5] The prevalence of varying editorial articles that provide opinions of the value of telemedicine[7] and its potential financial benefit,[8] coupled with telemedicine's incorporation into legislative initiatives,[9] show that as a practice, telemedicine is past the opinion-formation phase and has clearly accomplished the third stage, the decision to accept or reject the innovation, as evidenced by the ensuing prevalence of telemedicine programs.[5]

Perhaps this is best examined through the level of government approval that telemedicine receives. Government approval is necessary to regulate procedures and treatment methods; thus, government approval should shed light on the opinion of telemedicine and the decision to adopt or reject. For example, a program called BR Med-Connect at Our Lady of the Lake Regional Medical Center in Baton Rouge, Louisiana is a mobile telemedicine program linking the city's emergency medical services, such as ambulances, to hospital emergency rooms. The program sends live streaming video images from the ambulances through a Wi-Fi network downtown, which is

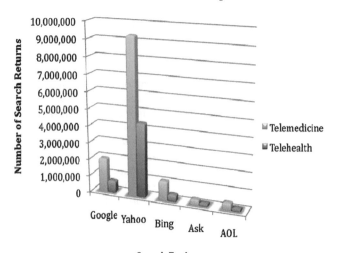

Fig. 4. Search engine results for "telemedicine" and "telehealth." (*Courtesy of* Arriaga R; with permission.)

supplemented by a 3G Evolution-Data Optimized (EV-DO) cellular network outside of downtown.[10] Baton Rouge is the second location in the country to implement this program. Tucson, Arizona in the Western region was the first, highlighting the unpredictable transference of telemedicine programs.[11] Thus, the local government has formulated a decision about telemedicine and made a decision to accept the innovation.

Accomplishment of the fourth phase of the innovation adoption process, execution or the active gathering of information and the implementation (regardless of the scale) of the program,[5] can be easily seen through a state-by-state search for telemedicine programs (**Fig. 5**). This search shows that each state has at least one telemedicine program operating; however, no single coordinated national telemedicine program exists.[4]

The fifth phase of the adoption decision process is confirmation. Confirmation refers to the decision to continue to use telemedicine or to enhance current programs.[5] It is in this stage that telemedicine currently resides. Programs, although plentiful, are constantly being evaluated for effectiveness and quality of care. For example, the Our Lady of the Lake – Hearing and Balance Center conducted a patient survey to gauge the satisfaction of patients seen through the telemedicine program versus those seen through a traditional office visit (Rabalais A, Arriaga MA. Patient satisfaction in a telemedicine neurotology program. Submitted for publication). The study found that patient satisfaction did not differ between the patient care delivery methods. Each program is unique unto itself and requires specific social engineering and business planning to successfully operate and meet a need.[12] Thus, telemedicine programs

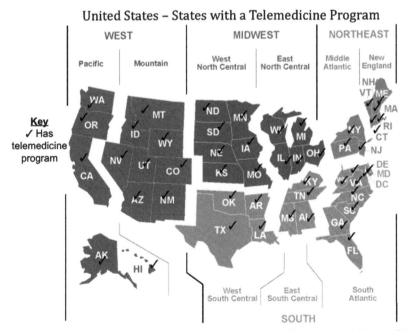

Fig. 5. Regional map of telemedicine regional assessment of the United States. (*From* Energy Information Administration. U.S. Census Regions and Divisions. Available at: http://www.eia.doe.gov/emeu/reps/maps/us_census.html. Accessed August 18, 2009.)

seem to diffuse via the reinvention theory described by Rogers.[5] This finding implies that no one program can be replicated exactly, but rather that programs must be modified for their individual contexts. This concept applies to individual programs that develop organically and to patented techniques implemented in different locations.

Despite the large presence and continued interest, telemedicine has yet to be fully incorporated into the United States health care delivery system. Each program is unique and developed for the individual health care center in which it is being integrated. As telemedicine programs arise in the United States, even if the new programs are emulating an existing program, the actual application will be somewhat different to conform to the individual needs of the location. However, until the programs are fully evaluated and a decision has been reached to accept or reject full-scale implementation of telemedicine throughout the health care delivery system, the programs remain in the confirmation stage of diffusion theory.

CLINICAL APPLICABILITY OF NEUROTOLOGY TELEMEDICINE
Manpower Considerations

The objective of a telemedicine program is to connect patients with providers when the availability of needed providers at the patient location is limited. Although natural disaster and educational applications are considered separately later in this article, current manpower predictions for otolaryngology and neurotology suggest that the demand will outstrip the supply of specialists, even before considering recent legislative changes potentially increasing economic/insurance access to physicians. Telemedicine represents an important potential remedy to this need/supply mismatch. Through extending the availability of specialty services to locations without a specialist, availability to specialty care is enhanced. These "satellite" strategies to remote locations can assure accurate screening evaluations at remote locations, with on-site subspecialty treatments in highly selected cases refractory to remote approaches. The American Academy of Otolaryngology has specifically included telemedicine as one potential solution to the impending shortage of otolaryngologists.[13,14] Community recognition of the potential value of these services is even being recognized in national[15] and local business journals.[16]

Telemedicine in the Aftermath of a Natural Disaster

Telemedicine's unique capabilities to connect professionals and patients are highlighted in the special crisis of a natural disaster. One of the coauthors (DN) summarizes the special role of telemedicine in maintaining the LSU otolaryngology department in the following personal essay:

> In August 2005, Hurricane Katrina decimated the coastal regions of Louisiana and Mississippi. Some of the most catastrophic storm-related flooding occurred in the densely populated area of metropolitan New Orleans. At least 1,836 deaths were attributed to the storm, and more than 70% of the city of New Orleans was inundated with flood waters, in some areas as much as 11 feet deep. Because New Orleans is partly below sea level and dependent on a levee system that failed in multiple places, the floodwaters persisted for many weeks. Hundreds of thousands of people who evacuated were prohibited from returning to their homes for several months, and those who remained in the city, or returned early on (in the sweltering late summer heat and humidity), were mostly living in primitive circumstances, with a desperate paucity of resources as basic as food, water, and electricity.
> Healthcare services were severely impacted. Wind damage and flooding from Katrina forced the closure of the majority of New Orleans' hospitals, and the

few that remained open were overwhelmed with patients in need of scarce resources. This included not only those suffering from storm-related injuries, infections and dehydration, but also many patients with chronic conditions who had lost access to medications, regular treatments, or life-saving interventions such as hemodialysis.

Understandably, in the aftermath of this desperate scenario, the provision of highly specialized healthcare services was severely limited. The widespread flooding had made much of the city uninhabitable, and many healthcare professionals and support personnel simply had nowhere to live. With doctors and nurses in short supply, hospitals struggled to provide even basic services, and as a result, subspecialty care was almost nonexistent.

Shortages of healthcare workers persisted for many months after the initial disaster. During the first year after Katrina, recruiting new physicians to the region was a daunting task. This was especially true in otolaryngology. While many of the region's general otolaryngologists had served at the forefront of emergency care and rescue operations, patients who had complex or unusual ENT [ear, nose, and throat] problems requiring tertiary referral had very few options.

With specialty physician manpower in such short supply, traditional face-to-face delivery of services was difficult, and at times impossible. Prior to Katrina, the Louisiana State University Health Sciences Center's Department of Otolaryngology-Head and Neck Surgery had conducted telemedicine-based patient care operations dating back to the early 1990's, mainly providing service to rural areas or incarcerated populations of the state's prison system. After Katrina, in the months when the New Orleans-based Department was forced to operate from satellite locations in nearby cities of Baton Rouge and Lafayette, it became logical to revisit the telemedicine strategy.

Based on the Department's prior telemedicine experience, and in conjunction with Dr. Moises A. Arriaga's own personal experience with neurotology consultations delivered via telemedicine in other areas of the country, it became obvious that the needs of neurotology patients in our region could be well served using a telemedicine delivery system. Thus, a telemedicine neurotology system was born of necessity.

In parallel with the pressing need for patient care, there was an equally compelling need for re-establishing medical education programs for Louisiana's medical students and residents. Just as Katrina had forced closure of multiple hospitals in the New Orleans area, it had also forced displacement of medical trainees into temporary assignments at schools and residency programs in other cities, including many programs nationwide, who had generously responded to the urgency of the disaster. While these arrangements were extremely helpful in the short term, it was clear that Louisiana's medical education system also needed to be rebuilt. Telemedicine played an integral part in our educational plans as well. Initially we relied on teleconferencing simply as a means to provide didactic lectures, and as we gained more experience with it, we expanded it as a means for case presentations, resident evaluations, and educational demonstrations of surgical techniques.

In the months and years after the 2005 Katrina disaster, we have come to appreciate the exceptional power of telemedicine as a tool for both patient care and medical education. Elsewhere in this monograph, the fine points of telemedicine implementation, patient acceptance, costs, reimbursement issues, technical limitations and other practical considerations will be presented in detail, along with references and suggested readings. From a broad perspective, however, what we have learned is quite simple: telemedicine can play a very effective role in subspecialty patient care as well as high quality education.

We have objectively studied the "outcomes" of our telemedicine programs and have been extremely pleased at what we have seen. Patients who have received neurotology consultations and treatment via telemedicine have expressed levels *of satisfaction that are comparable to, and in some cases better than, the traditional model of one-on-one same-site care [Rabalais A, Arriaga MA. Patient satisfaction in a telemedicine neurotology program. Submitted for publication]. We believe this is attributable in part to the appeal of the "high-tech" approach, but also to the fact that the patient is receiving expert attention from several professionals simultaneously, including the nurse practitioner conducting the exam, the audiologist obtaining the physiologic data, and the physician who interprets the findings and makes recommendations. One cannot over-emphasize the importance of having a dedicated team of such professionals who are focused on furnishing an uncompromising, high-quality service.*

Educationally, we found that telemedicine greatly expanded our ability to give medical trainees exposure to didactic material, technical training, and direct patient care. We actively included the telemedicine clinic experience in residents' schedules and made them responsible for some of the services; this not only led to additional patient satisfaction but also furnished us with a new tool for documenting and evaluating residents' performance – an increasingly important requirement in meeting their ultimate training requirements. As for didactic outcomes, in the first year of implementation of a teleconference-driven curriculum, our LSU residents scored in the 90th percentile nationwide on the standardized Otolaryngology Training Exam (OTE). Obviously this success is not only due to telemedicine, and cannot have been possible without extremely dedicated faculty and residents, but if anything it signifies that a teleconference-based Otolaryngology curriculum is, at the very least, workable.

Neurotology, the subject of this paper, is perhaps uniquely suited to a telemedicine delivery system. The use of high-resolution video-otoscopes, video-microscopy, and video-transmission of objective visual information including audiograms, vestibular test results, and CT and MR scans, for example, are all crucial elements in a good neurotological evaluation. But how adaptable is the technology for other otolaryngology patients? Our early experience suggests that it is also quite good. While it is not (yet) practical to use telemedicine equipment to transmit an objective sense of tactile findings, such as the palpation of an enlarged neck node, tongue base lesion, or thyroid mass, it is certainly easy to remotely transmit results of an ultrasound exam or CT/MR scan of such disease. Other components of the general ENT/head and neck exam are quite straightforward, including video exam of the external appearance of the head, face and neck, inspection of the oral cavity and nose with appropriate illumination, and video rhinoscopy as well as laryngoscopy. We are actively incorporating general otolaryngology services into our telemedicine programs. Given the projected manpower limits in Otolaryngology subspecialties in the next decade, along with political and socio-economic constraints that make subspecialty care challenging, we believe that telemedicine will continue to be an essential tool for the future.

Telemedicine Considerations in Cochlear Implantation

Although candidate evaluation for cochlear implantation uses many of the standard tools of neurotology telemedicine, remote intraoperative testing and remote implant programming are increasing applications of neurotology telemedicine. For candidate evaluation, communication can be an obstructing treatment barrier. Because the patients are candidates for implantation, amplification for louder volume and use of an frequency modulated trainer are not reasonable options. Instead, a sign language interpreter or closed captioning is necessary. In the authors' experience, the physician can type questions and answers to the patient's questions using a standard word processing computer program. Through selecting a large font, the patient and family can see the text on the large-screen TV/computer monitor. This technique can supplement the role of the sign interpreter; however, many patients find that the real-time typing communication is more spontaneous and lends itself to true interaction, joking, and spontaneity.

An important trend in cochlear implantation is remote integrity/impedance testing and remote programming. After surgical placement of a cochlear implant, confirmation of the electrode functionality is accomplished through connecting a magnet interface and running a computer-based electronic function assessment. Generally this is accomplished with an audiologist in the operating room; however, this approach commits an audiologist to accompanying the surgical team in the operating room. The ability to accomplish the integrity testing without the audiologist being physically present the operating room is an important telemedicine application that improves the efficiency of neurotologic care.

The authors' team has successfully applied commercially available software for remote control of a computer in another location through an Internet program. The opportunity to improve the quality of intraoperative cochlear implantation care through remote consultation with experts from the manufacturer or other cochlear implant centers is now unlimited by geographic location.[17] Another telemedicine application in cochlear implantation is remote programming of the cochlear implant. In this fashion, the patient can be in any location with Internet access and the programming audiologist has full control of the programming software. Simultaneous use of the videoconferencing software by the remote expert audiologist and the patient at another location allows the audiologist to be certain that the device has been properly placed, activated, and adjusted. This approach has already allowed international activation and programming of cochlear implants for patients in remote locations.[18]

Our Lady of the Lake Regional Medical Center–LSU Neurotology Telemedicine Program

The detailed structure and outcomes of the Our Lady of the Lake Regional Medical Center–LSU Neurotology Telemedicine Program are discussed elsewhere (Rabalais A, Arriaga MA. Patient satisfaction in a telemedicine neurotology program. Submitted for publication).[19] During the initial year, a fully equipped neurotology clinic was staffed by the neurotologist (MA) on-site for 1 week per month and through telemedicine connection 3 weeks per month. Equipment included an audiometer, a tympanometer, and a sound booth; electrophysiologic equipment for audiometric brainstem response, electrocochleography, and vestibular evoked myogenic response; a rotational chair; equipment for computerized posturography, autorotation vestibular testing, and visual nystagmogram; and infrared video goggles for nystagmus recording. The specific telemedicine equipment included a codec (Tandberg Intern, Tandberg, Tandberg Inc, [part of Cisco Corporation] San Jose, CA, USA), video endoscope adaptable to codec, microscope camera adaptable to codec, and digital converter for films or paper data transmission for codec, and infrared video goggles with a codec adapter. The initial staff included a full-time nurse practitioner, full-time audiologist licensed practical nurse, medical assistant, medical secretary, and office manager. Additional physician support was provided by the full-time presence of the collaborating neurosurgeon and the head and neck division of the otolaryngology department within the same office building. However, use of these supporting physicians has not been required for clinical emergencies.

Clinical pathways as standardized tools for evaluation have been a critical component of the telemedicine program. Specifically, when patients are scheduled for an evaluation, their assessment and testing are arranged based on required tests for each diagnosis according to preestablished algorithms. In this fashion, standardized objective data are available for review during the clinical visit. A typical patient visit occurs in the afternoon after the nurse practitioner visit and audiologic testing are completed in the morning. The results of the tests and the initial nurse practitioner evaluation are sent via fax to the neurotologist for interpretation during the patient visit. The patient is then evaluated via teleconference with the nurse practitioner and medical assistant present. After the history is completed, a physical examination is completed with the assistance of the teleconference unit, with the neurotologist in Pittsburgh and the patient and remainder of the team in Baton Rouge. A full neurotologic evaluation is completed, including a full head and neck examination and otologic examination with microscope and endoscope, tuning fork examination, nystagmus evaluation, gait assessment, Romberg test, Fukuda stepping test, and cranial nerve examination. The neurotologist and patient review the images as they are simultaneously shown on a large-screen TV for the patient and clinical team in Baton Rouge and on a computer screen for the neurotologist in Pittsburgh. Once the evaluation is completed, the diagnosis is discussed and short computer slide (PowerPoint) presentations are reviewed outlining the pathology and treatment options for the patient.

During the first year of the program, more than 800 patient visits were performed through telemedicine with 140 surgeries. No patient visits were incomplete because of technical issues with the equipment. Of the surgeries performed during the first year, 40% of the patients first met the neurotologist in person on the day of the surgery, because the clinical evaluation and informed consent process had occurred through telemedicine. Clinical outcomes analysis using validated outcome measurement tools is underway; however, no difference has yet been seen in clinical outcome. From the standpoint of patient satisfaction, the results have been surprising. A recent formal evaluation of the satisfaction data obtained from quality improvement data has shown that patient satisfaction is actually higher for telemedicine than on-site visits for the full spectrum of parameters, including "sense of connecting with the physician," "availability of the physician," "access to the physician," and "comfort with the setting." These surveys also indicated that the telemedicine neurotology experience significantly exceeded the patients' expectations of the process.

ADMINISTRATIVE ISSUES FOR NEUROTOLOGY TELEMEDICINE

The practice management perspectives of any health care delivery method are vital to its success. Medical licensure for the physician at both the physician location and the patient location is the safest legal strategy. Some states permit licensing exceptions for certain high-need specialties or in times of natural disaster. Anyone contemplating these activities should specifically evaluate their own state's requirements. Similarly with malpractice, coverage at the location of patient care is essential; however, the provider should evaluate their standing with their malpractice carrier. Third-party insurance coverage for medical visits was a specific concern during implementation of the Our Lady of the Lake – LSU program. The authors' reimbursement experts had meetings with the private insurers and government insurance programs. The private insurers accepted the visits as regular physician services and reimbursed accordingly. Although Medicare has specific provisions encouraging the development of telemedicine in medically underserved areas, Baton Rouge did not qualify geographically for this status. Accordingly, the visits have been coded as mid-level provider visits for Medicare, because the nurse practitioner performed a separate history and examination. The Medicare issue is one expected to be remedied soon.

Although the initial program was a necessary step to maintain clinical services and the otolaryngology residency after Hurricane Katrina, the benefits have extended far beyond the initial intent, including identifying a practical technique to extend services to underserved areas and potentially help alleviate the pending shortage of otolaryngologists.

FUTURE APPLICATIONS

The next level in neurotologic applications of telemedicine parallels the wider diffusion of telemedicine and its acceptance in medicine in general. The principal objective of the authors' system is to use telemedicine to ease integration with other specialties within the medical center and to extend the reach to underserved areas through telemedicine-facilitated satellite offices.

REFERENCES

1. Smith A, Bensink M, Armfield N, et al. Telemedicine and rural health care applications. J Postgrad Med 2005;51(4):286–93.
2. Eikelboom RH, Mbao MN, Coates HL, et al. Validation of tele-otology to diagnose ear disease in children. Int J Pediatr Otorhinolaryngol 2005;69(6):739–44.
3. Alaskan Federal Health Care Access NEtwork. Telemedicine Equipment. Available at: http://www.afhcan.org/. Accessed June 5, 2010.
4. Arriaga RY. An exploration of the diffusion of telemedicine and the impact of differing healthcare delivery systems: a US and Australian comparison [dissertation]. Fife, Scotland, United Kingdom: University of St. Andrews; 2009.
5. Rogers E. Diffusion of innovations. 4th edition. New York: The Free Press; 1995.
6. Cisco Corporation. The Doctor is in. Available at: http://videolounge.cisco.com/video/the-doctor-is-in/. Accessed April 25, 2009.
7. Dickson H. Hospital's telemedicine program helps save local woman's life. Sequoyah County Times Web site. Available at: http://www.sequoyahcountytimes.com/pages/full_story/push?article-Hospital's+telemedicine+program+helps+save+local+woman's+life%20&id=3112758&instance=home_news_bullets. Accessed August 17, 2009.
8. Bulford T. Profit from an ageing population. Money Week Web site. Available at: http://www.moneyweek.com/investment-advice/profit-from-an-ageing-population-14748.aspx. Accessed August 17, 2009.
9. House bill report: SHB 1529. Available at: http://apps.leg.wa.gov/documents/billdocs/2009-10/Pdf/Bill%20Reports/House/1529-S%20HBR%20PL%2009.pdf. Accessed August 16, 2009.
10. Baton Rouge launches EMS telemedicine program. EMSWorld Web site. Available at: http://www.publicsafety.com/web/online/ED-industry-Wite/Baton-Rouge-Launches-EMS-Telemedicine-Program/33$9279. Accessed August 17, 2009.
11. Ambulance service uses Wi-Fi network for telemedicine. H&HN Web site. Available at: http://www.hhnmag.com/hhnmag_app/jsp/articledisplay.jsp?dcrpath=HFMMAGAZINE/Article/data/06JUN2009/0906HFM_upfront_information&domain=HFMMAGAZINE. Accessed August 16, 2009.
12. Grigsby J, Rigby M, Hiemstra A, et al. The diffusion of telemedicine. Telemed J E Health 2002;8:79–94.
13. Workforce shortage gap: not expected to be closed in the coming decade. American Academy of Otolaryngology – Head and Neck Surgery Web site. Available at: http://aao-365.ascendeventmedia.com/highlight.aspx?id=82&p=4. Accessed August 13, 2011.
14. Henkel G. Filling the gap: strategies for addressing the otolaryngology workforce shortage. ENT Today Web site. Available at: http://www.enttoday.org/details/

article/554349/Fill_the_Gap_Strategies_for_addressing_the_otolaryngology_workforce_shortage.html. Accessed August 13, 2011.

15. Freudenheim M. The doctor will see you now, please log on. Available at: http://www.nytimes.com/2010/05/30/business/30telemed.html. Accessed June 11, 2010.

16. Brown T. Dial-a-Doctor. BusinessReport.com; Available at: http://www.businessreport.com/news/2010/mar/08/dial–doctor-hlcr1/?print. Accessed August 13, 2011.

17. McElveen J, Blackburn E, Green D, et al. Remote programming of cochlear implants: a telecommunications model. Otol Neurotol 2010;31(7):1035–40.

18. Ramos A, Rodriguez C, Martinez-Beneyto P, et al. Use of telemedicine in the remote programming of Cochlear Implantation. Acta Otolaryngol 2009;129(5): 533–40.

19. Arriaga MA, Nuss DW, Scrantz K, et al. Telemedicine-assisted neurotology in Post Katrina, Southeast Louisiana. Otol Neurotol 2010;31(3):524–7.

Telehealth and Humanitarian Assistance in Otolaryngology

Kelly L. Groom, MD[a], Mitchell J. Ramsey, MD[a],*,
James E. Saunders, MD[b]

KEYWORDS

- Telehealth • Telemedicine • Humanitarian aid
- Humanitarian assistance • Otolaryngology

Key Points: HUMANITARIAN ASSISTANCE IN OTOLARYNGOLOGY THROUGH TELEHEALTH

- Worldwide many underserved regions have a large burden of head and neck disease. In many of these region there are insufficient specialists to provide care.

- Otolaryngology as a specialty has a strong history of humanitarian involvement to help meet the needs of these regions.

- Telehealth uses asynchronous or synchronous technology to provide health services over a distance and is an evolving tool that can enhance humanitarian efforts.

- Simple everyday technology, such as e-mail and image store and forwarding, is already used successfully to provide medical care to underserved areas worldwide.

- Evolving telehealth issues include medicolegal clarification, international regulations, cost, and advancing technology. Most successful telehealth programs result from humanitarian partnerships based on collaboration, planning, and persistence.

- Telehealth is an evolving field with tremendous potential, but further research is necessary to establish its efficacy, safety, and impact.

The views expressed in this article are those of the authors and do not reflect the official policy or position of the Department of the Army, Department of Defense, or the U.S. Government.
[a] Division of Otolaryngology, Tripler Army Medical Center, 1 Jarrett White Road, Tripler AMC, Honolulu, HI 96859, USA
[b] Department of Otolaryngology, Dartmouth Medical Center, One Medical Center Drive, Lebanon, NH 03756, USA
* Corresponding author. Otolaryngology Service, Tripler Army Medical Center, 1 Jarrett White Road, Tripler AMC, Honolulu, HI 96859.
E-mail address: mitchell.ramsey@us.army.mil

Otolaryngol Clin N Am 44 (2011) 1251–1258
doi:10.1016/j.otc.2011.08.002
0030-6665/11/$ – see front matter Published by Elsevier Inc.

Humanitarian efforts include a broad range of measures to assist underserved populations. These efforts can include needs assessment, environmental projects, infrastructure improvement, public health education, and medical services. Many otolaryngologists are familiar with the medical aspects of humanitarian activities (HAs). Several actively participate in clinical field missions, and some have been involved in policy development, education, and promotion of otolaryngology services at the global level. Most physicians involved with HAs have a tremendous sense of gratification and satisfaction from helping the less fortunate. However, most will also readily attest to the daunting clinical need and frustration associated with the inability to accomplish more. Regardless of the setting or location, the need for humanitarian medical care is extensive, and the need to augment and expand HA is widely recognized. Telehealth, through the use of information and communication technology (ICT), is an obvious and practical tool to achieve this goal.

For the purposes of this article, "telehealth" refers to any field of health care that uses telecommunication to transmit medical information across distances, and would include a means of providing professional and public education and patient care. Telemedicine is one aspect of telehealth that generally refers to the clinical aspect and includes consultative services. In HAs, telemedicine allows patients in underserved regions to receive specialty consultation.

World Health Organization (WHO) Director General, Dr Hiroshi Nakajima, said in 1997, "Developing an adequate and affordable telecommunication infrastructure can help to close the gap among the haves and the have-nots in health care." The potential of telehealth to reduce inequalities in health care is immense but remains underdeveloped. Providing care and consultation at a distance using ICT is an enterprise that continues to expand and develop in stride with developing technology and changing policies. This article explores some of the important features of telehealth use in humanitarian projects and provides examples of successful applications.

OTOLARYNGIC BURDEN OF DISEASE

A large need for otolaryngology services exists in the developing world. This is because of a extensive disease burden and a paucity of trained otolaryngologists. Major contributors to higher disease incidences include environmental factors, nutritional deficiencies, limited public health measures, and behavioral risk factors. Of equal significance is the limited availability of otolaryngology specialists. Most developing countries have little or no capacity to provide subspecialty care, such as otolaryngology, audiology, or speech pathology. For instance, in Africa the average number of otolaryngologists per 100,000 people is 0.11 compared with 3.1 (in 2004) in the United States.[1]

Examples illustrating the burden of otolaryngic disease include chronic otitis media, oral and oropharyngeal cancer, and thyroid disease. The WHO estimates that chronic otitis media is a major contributor to acquired hearing loss in developing countries, with the worldwide global burden of illness from chronic suppurative otitis media involving 65 to 330 million individuals. Of these individuals, 60% (39–200 million) have significant hearing impairment, meaning that chronic suppurative otitis media may contribute more than half the global burden of hearing impairment, and eliminating it can potentially reduce the global burden by four-fifths.[2]

Two-thirds of the worldwide burden of oral and oropharyngeal cancer is from developing nations. In many regions, such as Sri Lanka, India, Pakistan, and Bangladesh, oral cancer is the most common cancer in men. Higher cancer rates and poorer outcomes are correlated with more disadvantaged populations. The 5-year survival rate for oral cavity and oropharyngeal cancers in these countries is as low as 50%. This low survival rate is caused by multiple factors, including delayed detection and decreased access to care.[3]

Surgical thyroid disease represents another condition often managed by otolaryngologists with a high global burden. Iodine deficiency resulting in thyroid goiter was estimated to affect nearly 10% of the world's population (536 million people worldwide).[4,5] Prevention with iodine replacement is critical, but surgical management is often beneficial for large existing goiters. Randolph[6] published an excellent review with a more complete picture of the global distribution, impact, and management of thyroid disease.

OTOLARYNGOLOGY HUMANITARIAN EFFORTS

Because of limited resources, most developing countries focus their efforts on public health, preventive measures, and primary health care needs. Therefore, the tremendous need for specialty care is often deemphasized or overlooked. The high otolaryngologic disease burden and insufficient number of trained specialists has led many otolaryngologists within these countries and from the developed world to reach out and provide assistance to these underserved populations. As specialists, the role of otolaryngologists in HA is typically to provide direct patient care and consultation, but often they also act as consultants in education, training, and policy development. Direct patient care may occur within a focused otolaryngology mission or as a component of a multidisciplinary team.

Otolaryngologists specialize in the surgical and medical management of head and neck disorders. Therefore, they can play a critical role in the development of public health programs, allied health services, and educational programs for these diseases. As a specialty, otolaryngology has a strong history of humanitarian involvement. The Humanitarian Efforts Committee of the American Academy of Otolaryngology Head and Neck Surgery Foundation (AAO-HNSF) was founded in 1985 and serves to support the humanitarian activities of its members and to advocate for programs that improve the prevention and treatment of otolaryngologic disorders within under-resourced areas of the United States and abroad. More information is available at http://www.entnet.org/Community/public/Becoming-Involved.cfm.

TELEHEALTH AND INFORMATION AND COMMUNICATION TECHNOLOGY

Telehealth is a spectrum of health services conducted over a distance using ICT to support clinical health care, patient and professional health-related education, public health, and health administration. Telehealth is conducted using two basic methods: store and forward (asynchronous) or real-time (synchronous). The method chosen depends on many factors, including the type (eg, documents, images, video), quantity and nature of information being transmitted, the urgency of the transmission, local conditions and capabilities, security, and privacy. Hartnett[7] identified three essential components of a telehealth system: personnel, technology, and perseverance, and provides an excellent review of the telemedicine technology and more insight into the details of a successful system. In terms of technology, a telemedicine system has three basic categories: acquisition equipment, telecommunications transmission equipment, and reception and display equipment.

Acquisition equipment usually includes computers and methods to digitize information, such as scanners. It also includes equipment for acquiring images, video or audio and the collection of other clinically relevant diagnostic information. Transmission ICT equipment may include telephone lines, cellular phones, Internet, and satellite transmission. Decreasing costs and easier applications are allowing telehealth infrastructures to become more feasible. However, significant barriers remain, limiting the integration of these technologies into daily health care practice. Thoughtful consideration should be given to the ICT setup that depends on Internet access, because according to statistics published by the International Telecommunications Union, only 15.8% of households in developing nations currently have this access.[8] Satellite telecommunication technologies have advanced and are now available worldwide, but they remain expensive.

Although the technological details of a telehealth setup are not the focus of this article, some broad principles should be understood. The technologies best suited for use in humanitarian aid must be appropriate, durable, simple, and affordable. First and foremost, the technologic application must be appropriate to the local infrastructure. For example, pursuing remote robotic surgery in an isolated African village is not feasible. In their article entitled "The Seven Sins of Humanitarian Medicine," Welling and colleagues[9] described failing to match technology to local needs and abilities as one of the cardinal mistakes in humanitarian aid. Second, the modalities used must be durable enough to withstand transportation to their destination and variable climate conditions, including possible extremes in temperature or humidity. Dry, safe storage must be available for computers, cameras, and telephones. Simple repair of these devices may not be feasible in some environments. The technology used must also be simple to apply and easy to teach. Many individuals from developed countries have integrated technology into their daily lives, but this may not be the case for people in developing regions of the world. Finally, cost will always be a significant, if not the limiting, factor in the integration of telehealth into HAs. Although the cost of many forms of technology is decreasing (ie, the cost of the average computer in the United States has declined 90% in the past 10 years) the price of satellite time, cellular networks, Internet connectivity, and major infrastructure endeavors remains a real burden for countries most in need of humanitarian aid. Telehealth technology and infrastructure vary greatly among locations. However, in many developing regions, basic ICT infrastructures exist and can be integrated with specialized medical equipment to augment humanitarian efforts.

TELEHEALTH HUMANITARIAN EFFORTS

The size, complexity, and success of a telehealth program can vary dramatically and depends on the regional infrastructure, resources and goals of the organizations using the telehealth applications. In small-scale humanitarian projects, telehealth applications allow for communication in between missions. For example, e-mail or other store and forward communication can facilitate postoperative care, identify new patients for future missions, provide consultations, and enhance education. In larger-scale HA missions, such as those involving academic institutions or hospitals, the telehealth applications are more comprehensive, subject to more regulation and formal agreements, and better supported. The success of telehealth in HA relies on collaboration, planning, and prioritizing regardless of the level. The Global Forum on Telemedicine in 2007[10] identified several focus areas to facilitate the advancement of global health care via telemedicine. Key initiatives would increase (1) dialog between HA organizations and technology stakeholders to facilitate the development and implementation of technology, (2) the development of programs to train health care workers to use telemedicine technology, and (3) procurement of satellite transmission at a reduced cost for medical and educational ventures.

Successful humanitarian telehealth programs often rely on telehealth partnerships. The telehealth partnership is a collaboration between organizations to expand care and services to the underserved. These partnerships can be large-scale government programs but can also be an academic collaboration between "sister" institutions. Frequently the partnerships are of a smaller scale, resulting from the work of just a few providers.

The book *Telehealth in the Developing World* by Wooten and colleagues[11] is an excellent source for practical, thriving telemedicine examples. This article only highlights a few of the many examples of successful use of humanitarian telehealth. The Children's National Medical Center (CNMC) in Washington, DC has partnered with regional and international hospitals (in Qatar, Iraq, Morocco, Uganda, and Germany) to provide long-distance medical care to children, mostly in the area of pediatric cardiology. Using asynchronous digital echocardiograms and live video teleconferencing, cardiologists have expanded access to care for children with heart disease. The CNMC has also used the same technology to host distance education programs and live video teleconferencing presentations to include hospital grand rounds in Iraq and Morocco.

In South America, the Ecuadorian telehealth network has established connections between the Universedad Technologica Equinoccial and remote communities in the jungle and the Galapagos for the purpose of medical consultation. The Ecuadorian Air Force donated broadband satellite connectivity throughout the country to facilitate knowledge sharing and medical education.

The Swinfen Charitable Trust is an organization that provides store and forward equipment to medical providers in developing countries. More than 150 facilities in 50 countries benefit from this program. Medical Missions for Children is an organization that provides diagnostic consultations between partnering physicians and patients in remote locations in 100 countries via its telemedicine outreach program.

TELEHEALTH HUMANITARIAN ACTIVITIES IN OTOLARYNGOLOGY

The otolaryngology community has several exceptional individuals and organizations conducting sustained high-impact humanitarian care incorporating telehealth into clinical care or educational activities. The literature describing these efforts, however, is limited. Many individuals involved in these endeavors choose to channel their energies into their programs instead of writing about them. The examples, which follow, illustrate some of the ways telehealth has been incorporated into HAs.

The Pacific Island Health Care Program (PIHCP) is a telemedicine program that provides subspecialty medical consultation and care to insular nations of the South Pacific. The massive Pacific region is an area with many extremely remote locations, making the delivery of and access to care very challenging. This program uses a secure Web site for asynchronous health care, allowing remote physicians to consult specialists at Tripler Army Medical Center (TAMC), a tertiary Department of Defense Hospital. A Web site was designed to provide store and forward consultation (**Fig. 1**). Participants received computers, digital cameras, and scanners, which enable them to exchange information and communicate with specialists at TAMC. Detailed patient information, such as pertinent history and physical elements, laboratory values, radiographic studies, and photographs, can be transmitted to the appropriate specialist. A treatment recommendation is then promptly returned to the remote provider. Participants in the PICHP include Guam, Commonwealth of Marianna Islands, American Samoa, Republic of Marshall Islands, Federated States of Micronesia (Yap, Kosrae, Pohnpei, Chuuk), and the Republic of Palau. Patients are

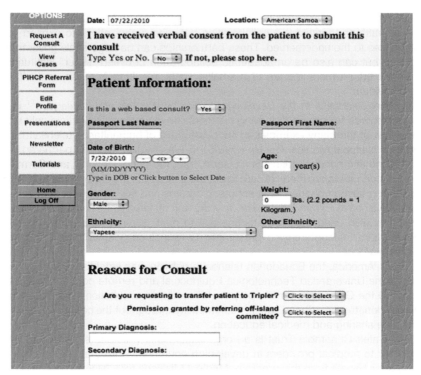

Fig. 1. Pacific island health care referral Web site.

referred for care in all specialties. The otolaryngology-head and neck service has extensive involvement and receives many referrals each year for complicated head and neck cancer and advanced chronic ear disease. Since its inception the PICHP has received over 3000 referrals. The PIHCP has been of tremendous benefit to graduate medical education, the medical staff, and of course the recipients of care in the South Pacific. It represents a successful joint humanitarian and telemedicine program and serves as a model for remote subspecialty consultation. The PIHCP allows for consultative services using simple technology and is a very cost-effective means to increase access to care for an underserved population.

As an extension of the PICHP, subspecialty medical teams deploy from TAMC to Micronesia to provide onsite care and consultation. One of these teams provides otolaryngology and audiology care. Palau is a remote republic that does not have a population large enough to support specialties such as otolaryngology or audiology. However, because Palau has a high incidence of chronic otitis media, itinerant otolaryngology consultants have provided treatment for many decades. The TAMC team conducts direct clinical and surgical care at local facilities. After departure, follow-up care involves the PIHCP Web site integrating telehealth to provide support between visits. Audiologists are part of the team and have assisted in establishing improved diagnostic capabilities and a newborn hearing screening program. The next phase of support has the goal of implementing amplification services and remote audiologic support.

Many humanitarian organizations incorporate telehealth to some degree, often developing creative solutions to a particular need. One outreach organization, Global ENT

Outreach, focuses on diseases of the ear and has a strong educational emphasis. They have assisted with training programs on hearing loss, use of hearing aids, and clinical management of chronic otitis media, and even have established regional temporal bone laboratories. A creative use of telehealth to augment its educational program is a journal club conducted between consultants and colleagues in Pnom Penh, Cambodia. Articles and a presentation are distributed via e-mail, then the journal club is conducted in real-time using Skype, a software application that allows users to make videoconferencing calls over the Internet (Richard Wagner, personal communication, 2010).

Another humanitarian group focusing on cleft lip and palate missions to Ecuador developed a telehealth solution to augment postoperative speech therapy. They created a virtual craniofacial team with capabilities to provide ongoing speech therapy remotely and occupational therapy using Web-based systems (Patrick Byrne, personal communication, 2010).

The Alaska experience, which is detailed elsewhere in this issue, is a superb demonstration of telehealth applications within otolaryngology. Kokesh and colleagues[12–14] have capitalized on telehealth to expand care and services to underserved populations. They have developed an asynchronous telemedicine program to augment their capabilities to provide subspecialty consultation and care. Their multiple publications validate the efficacy and cost-effectiveness of telehealth.

The AAO-HNSF AcademyU is an online educational resource for providers that allows users to participate in learning activities and keep track of continuing medical education. In an effort to make this online resource available to international colleagues, the AAO-HNSF recently began offering Internet subscriptions to nonmembers from foreign countries. Medical journals are available online to providers in developing countries through the WHO HINARI program, including more than 40 otolaryngology journals. Live International Otolaryngology Network is an online video teleconferencing network dedicated to otolaryngology. The site includes a regularly updated e-Library with a comprehensive collection of surgery videos, conferences, panel discussions, and virtual exhibition and conference halls.

SUMMARY

A tremendous burden of head and neck disease exists worldwide. Many practitioners within otolaryngology-head and neck surgery are committed to helping this underserved population. Awareness and interest in telehealth tools and technology is increasing, especially among residents who have grown up with the technology used in ICT and are very comfortable with its incorporation into health care. Several otolaryngology aid organizations incorporate ICT and telehealth into their efforts to expand the care they provide. The applications of remote diagnostic testing, specialty consultation, and provider and patient education can improve health care for underserved regions. Telehealth programs must be tailored to regional demands and constraints. Strong collaboration, thoughtful planning, and persistence are basic requirements for any program to be sustainable. In many underserved regions, an existing ICT infrastructure, dedicated personnel, and creative relationships have led to successful telehealth programs. Telehealth is still an emerging field and many efforts are underway to help facilitate partnerships. One very important way to promote telehealth use in HAs is to increase the data showing the quality of care, cost-effectiveness, and safety of telemedicine care. As ICT infrastructures expand, telecommunication costs decline, and telehealth policy evolves, the use of telehealth in underserved regions will continue to be a promising tool to augment care to patients most in need.

REFERENCES

1. Fagan JJ, Jacobs M. Survey of ENT services in Africa: need for a comprehensive intervention. Glob Health Action 2009;2:3.
2. WHO. Chronic suppurative otitis media: burden of illness and management options. Available at: http://www.who.int/pbd/deafness/activities/hearing_care/otitis_media.pdf. Accessed September 4, 2011.
3. Warnakulasuriya S. Global epidemiology of oral and oropharyngeal cancer. Oral Oncol 2009;45(4–5):309–31.
4. Delange FM. Iodine deficiency. In: Braverman L, Utiger RD, editors. The thyroid. 8th edition. Philadelphia: Lippincott Williams & Wilkins; 2000. p. 298–9.
5. The global burden of disease: 2004 update. World Health Organization Web site. Available at: http://www.who.int/healthinfo/global_burden_disease/2004_report_update/en/index.html. Accessed September 4, 2011.
6. Randolph GW. Surgery of the thyroid and parathyroid glands. Philadelphia: Elsevier Science; 2003.
7. Hartnett B. Telemedicine systems and telecommunications. J Telemed Telecare 2006;12:4–15.
8. ICT facts and figures: the world in 2010. International Telecommunications Union Web site. Available at: http://www.itu.int/ITU-D/ict/material/FactsFigures2010.pdf. Accessed July 26, 2011.
9. Welling DR, Ryan JM, Burris DG, et al. Seven sins of humanitarian medicine. World J Surg 2010;34:466–70.
10. Parks HS, Brown-Connolly NE, Bloch C, et al. Global forum on telemedicine; connecting the world through partnerships. Telemed J E Health 2008;14(4):389–95.
11. Wooten R, Patil N, Scott R, et al. Telehealth in the Developing World. IDRC, London: Royal Society of Medicine Press; 2009.
12. Kokesh J, Fergusun AS, Patricoski C. Telehealth in Alaska: delivery of heath care services from a specialist's perspective. Int J Circumpolar Health 2004;63(4):387–400.
13. Kokesh J, Ferguson AS, Patricoski C, et al. Digital images for postsurgical follow-up of tympanostomy tubes in remote Alaska. Otolaryngol Head Neck Surg 2008;139(1):87–93.
14. Kokesh J, Ferguson AS, Patricoski C, et al. Traveling an audiologist to provide otolaryngology care using store-and-forward telemedicine. Telemed J E Health 2009;15(8):758–63.

Successful Telemedicine Programs in Otolaryngology

Frank G. Garritano, MD, David Goldenberg, MD*

KEYWORDS

- Telemedicine • Teleconsultation • Telehealth • Otolaryngology
- Otoscopy • Alaska telemedicine • Queensland telemedicine

Telemedicine refers to the use of telecommunications technology to provide remote access to medical diagnosis and patient care. As technology has improved and the costs of using that technology have decreased, the promise of telemedicine and its potential to enhance the quality of care, improve efficiency, and reduce costs has grown significantly. The use of the Digital Imaging and Communications in Medicine (DICOM) imaging standard in radiology, for example, led to the widespread adoption of a telemedical approach to radiologic imaging and interpretation that has now become the standard of care. Historically, radiology, dermatology, psychiatry, and cardiology account for the most widespread use of telemedicine in the United States, but otolaryngology remains uniquely suited to the use of telemedicine. In addition to patient history and physical examination, many otolaryngologic diagnoses reflect information obtained from objective sources, such as tympanograms, audiometry, and telescopic and diagnostic imaging. These sources can be easily transmitted to allow for remote interpretation. Like many medical specialists, otolaryngologists are usually found in urban settings, making access to specialty care in remote and rural settings challenging. One promising use of telemedicine involves providing care to rural settings that would otherwise be difficult to provide in person, and this is a particular need that telemedicine is uniquely positioned to provide for.

TELEMEDICINE: STORE AND FORWARD VERSUS LIVE FEEDS

Telemedicine consultations commonly take one of 2 forms:

1. Live and interactive
2. Delayed

The authors have nothing to disclose.
Division of Otolaryngology–Head & Neck Surgery, Department of Surgery, Penn State Hershey Medical Center, 500 University Drive, Mail Code H091, Hershey, PA 17033-0850, USA
* Corresponding author.
E-mail address: dgoldenberg@hmc.psu.edu

The live and interactive method is intuitively appealing because it most closely approximates a real-life patient encounter; however, the use of a live consultation requires a level of coordination between the patient, referring physician, and specialist physician that makes this method of teleconsultation both more expensive and more challenging logistically.

The second form of telemedicine consultation is commonly known as store and forward. This involves the referring physician collecting and forwarding all of the relevant patient information, including history and imaging, to the consulting physician who then can review the data at a later time. One advantage of this type of consultation is that it does not require the physical presence of the referring physician or the patient (**Fig. 1**).

In 1997, Sclafani and colleagues[1] at the New York Eye and Ear Infirmary presented a study at the annual meeting of the American Academy of Otolaryngology - Head and Neck Surgery investigating the use of live and store-and-forward telemedicine in their otolaryngology practice. Patients were interviewed by a chief resident in otolaryngology who performed a relevant physical exam and flexible fiberoptic nasopharyngolaryngoscopy and who then presented his findings to 2 people: a locally available otolaryngologist and a remote otolaryngologist. Both the local and remote otolaryngologists were able to observe the interaction as well as a fiberoptic nasopharyngolaryngoscopy and to direct the chief resident. Afterward, another otolaryngologist, who was not present for the live encounter, was asked to review the electronic patient

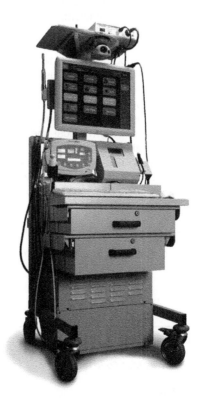

Fig. 1. A telemedicine cart used to collect information during a patient encounter for later review by a remote otolaryngologist using store-and-forward telemedicine. (Image *Courtesy of* the Alaska Native Tribal Health Consortium, Anchorage (AK); with permission.)

records. The investigators found concordance rates of 92% between the local and remote otolaryngologists (live videoconference) with a slightly lower concordance of 64% between the live physician and the delayed remote physician (store and forward). The investigators explain the diagnostic discordance seen with the store-and-forward remote physician as primarily the result of technical problems: color-shifting phenomenon, degraded video quality, and an insufficient quantity of high-quality images. Sclafani and colleagues[1] state that these are problems that are easily remedied by the capability of new technology to provide a greater number of higher-quality still and video images. They conclude that remote interactive tele-otolaryngology can be used to evaluate a range of patient complaints with a high degree of diagnostic reliability.[1]

TELEMEDICINE AND VIDEO OTOSCOPIC IMAGING

Otitis media is one of the most commonly encountered diagnoses in both pediatric and otolaryngologic practice, and the cost associated with the diagnosis and treatment of the disease is estimated to be in excess of 5.3 billion dollars per year.[2] Acute otitis media is the most common bacterial infection in children and is the most frequent indication for antimicrobial therapy in the pediatric population (**Fig. 2**). Patients who suffer from either recurrent acute otitis media or chronic otitis media are often treated with tympanostomy tube insertion, which is currently one of the most common procedures performed in children in the United States. After surgery, patients are seen in follow-up in the clinic to assess the patency of the tympanostomy tubes. This follow-up commonly occurs 1 month after surgery and at regular intervals thereafter. Because a significant proportion of the United States population lives in rural settings without nearby access to subspecialty surgical care, arranging follow-up for these patients can be challenging, which presents a unique opportunity for telemedicine to play a role in the postsurgical follow-up of patients with tympanostomy tubes.

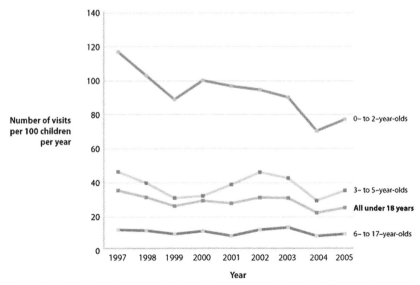

Fig. 2. Physician office visits resulting in a diagnosis of otitis media. The number of office visits per 100 children resulting in a diagnosis of otitis media, grouped by year and stratified by age group. (*Courtesy of* the National Institutes of Health.)

To establish a role for video otoscopy in providing telemedical care, it is important to ensure that video otoscopy is an accurate form of data gathering and that it provides reproducible results when images are reviewed by different practitioners. In 2003, Patricoski and colleagues[3] of the Alaska Native Medical Center addressed this question in a study examining whether the results of still images of the tympanic membrane were comparable with in-person microscopic examination. They selected 40 patients who had previously undergone tympanostomy tube placement, had them independently examined by 2 otolaryngologists, and had imaging done using a video otoscope (**Fig. 3**). The examining otolaryngologists reviewed the images 6 and 12 weeks later and the investigators compared their diagnostic concordance using κ statistics. Patricoski and colleagues[3] found that intraprovider concordance rates were between 85% and 99% for physical examination findings and between 79% and 85% for diagnosis. They conclude that store-and-forward video otoscopy may be an appropriate method of following tympanostomy tubes after placement.

Studies in the Literature

A study published in 2004 examined the use of video otoscopy to assess and diagnose middle ear disease. Aronzon and colleagues[4] from the University of Pennsylvania compared groups of medical students, internal medicine residents, and attending and resident otolaryngologists who were presented with a set of matched tympanograms and photographs of the tympanic membrane obtained through video otoscopy. Subjects were asked to differentiate between a normal-appearing and abnormal-appearing membrane and to make a diagnosis of middle ear disease based on the imaging. The investigators reported that the sensitivity of diagnosis by attending otolaryngologists using tympanograms and photographs was equal to the sensitivity of diagnosis achieved with the operating microscope. The investigators concluded that video otoscopy technology can allow the expertise of a specialist to be extended to rural and underserved areas where specialists might not otherwise be available.[4]

A study in 2008 further developed the concept of using video otoscopy as a tool for clinical imaging of the tympanic membrane. Lundberg and colleagues[5] from Sweden studied 64 children aged 2 to 16 years with otalgia who presented to clinics in Sweden. The children had their tympanic membranes imaged using a video otoscope and had the images independently assessed by both an otolaryngologist and a general practitioner. The investigators analyzed overall image quality as well as quality of image-related components, such as focus, light, or composition. The investigators concluded that there was good overall agreement between examiners and that video otoscopy is a reliable technique in the clinical or research setting.[5] The investigators further pointed out that a potential advantage of digital imaging is that it may allow

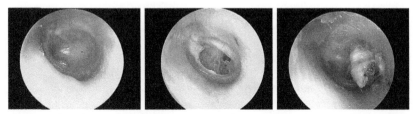

Fig. 3. Examples of images of the tympanic membrane obtained using a video otoscope. (Image *Courtesy of* the Alaska Native Tribal Health Consortium, Anchorage (AK); with permission.)

for more objective grading of the tympanic membrane and for retrospective review by independent examiners.[5]

In 2008, Kokesh and colleagues[6] published a study from Anchorage, Alaska detailing how they successfully made use of video otoscopy to allow for patient follow-up after tympanostomy tube insertion in remote areas of Alaska. They noted that American Indian and Alaskan native children have higher rates of otitis media and tympanostomy tube placement, but live in an environment that makes postsurgical follow-up challenging and expensive.[6] They used telemedicine to follow patients with tympanostomy tubes and examined the concordance between an in-person encounter and images of the tympanic membrane taken in remote village clinics. A similar study was done by Patricoski[3] in 2003 and is mentioned earlier; however, the 2003 study was performed in a controlled research environment and was not done in an authentic real-world clinical setting. Kokesh and colleagues[6] used community health aides and practitioners who performed video otoscopy in remote village clinics, in the same way that a telemedicine otolaryngology practice might operate. These images were then reviewed by an otolaryngologist. Between 1 and 7 days following their video otoscopic examination, the patients were flown to Maniilaq Health Center in Kotzebue for an otolaryngology clinic visit, where 2 otolaryngologists examined the patients using a Zeiss otology microscope. The video and microscopic otoscopic examinations were then evaluated for concordance.

The investigators in the 2008 Kokesh study examined a real-world practice environment using store-and-forward telemedicine with nonphysician health workers taking images of the tympanic membrane with no access to an operating microscope for ear cleaning.[6] The investigators found a high level of concordance between the image reviews and the in-person encounters, with 79% agreement between the remote and in-person encounters. Nineteen percent of all video otoscope images were rejected as being of poor or very poor quality. This finding was most commonly the result of poor focus leading to poor image quality or to cerumen or debris in the ear obstructing the field of view. In a real-life situation, these poor-quality images could easily be retaken on request, which led the investigators to conclude that high-quality digital images of the tympanic membrane can be obtained by a trained health aide in a rural setting, and that store-and-forward otoscopy can be used for tympanostomy tube follow-up in settings where the patient is located remotely from the specialist.[6]

SUCCESSFUL TELEMEDICINE PROGRAMS IN OTOLARYNGOLOGY
Alaskan Programs

Alaska has a land area of 1,517,733 km^2 (586,000 square miles) and a population density of 2.9 persons/km^2 (1.1 persons per square mile), which can make the delivery of specialty health care to remote areas challenging.[7] Seventy-five percent of Alaskan communities are not connected by road to the nearest hospital, and patients frequently travel great distances by air to see a provider, resulting in frequently missed appointments, high travel costs, and clinical deterioration while waiting to see an appropriate specialist.[8] Most of the state of Alaska is designated as a Health Professional Shortage Area,[9] and Alaska has the sixth lowest physician/population ratio in the nation.[10] Since 1999, the Ear, Nose, and Throat (ENT) department at Alaska Native Medical Center has been successfully using a telemedicine program to facilitate the care of patients living in remote areas. The remote consultation typically takes the form of a store-and-forward consultation, in which a clinical history, audiogram, images, tympanogram, and other patient information are reviewed remotely by an otolaryngologist who makes treatment and triage decisions to the referring provider.

In 2004, Kokesh and colleagues[8] from the Alaska Native Medical Center published an article detailing their success in implementing a telemedicine program in the Otolaryngology department at their facility. The investigators recognized that their traditional system for delivery of health care in remote areas of Alaska resulted in extremely long wait times, creating significant difficulty in triaging patients to determine who needed to be seen urgently. In addition, the process of traveling to see a specialist at their medical center was frequently expensive and, occasionally, even dangerous. They believed telemedicine could occupy a niche in their practice that would fulfill a clinical need.

The investigators published several studies determining the feasibility and efficacy of using video otoscopy in telemedicine, which are discussed earlier.[3,6] This work established the basis for the accuracy of diagnoses obtained via telemedical consultation. The investigators subsequently implemented a successful program for following patients after tympanostomy tube insertion using a store-and-forward telemedicine practice (**Fig. 4**).[3] The program has since expanded and the Alaska Native Medical Center is now able to receive telemedicine consultations from more than 200 remote sites in rural Alaska from several different sources, such as from small village clinics, from community health aides, from referring primary care doctors, or from rural hospitals.[8]

Change in Alaska telemedicine otolaryngology practice

In 2009, Kokesh and colleagues[8] published an article in which they described a change in their telemedicine otolaryngology practice. Patients who had a telemedicine visit were traditionally seen by specially trained nurses and other clinical staff who gathered the clinical history and the appropriate studies, such as a video otoscopic examination, audiogram, tympanogram, and other relevant documents. In 2009, the investigators used a specially trained audiologist to travel to remote areas and gather the necessary information relevant for a telemedicine consultation. They hypothesized that, because audiologists had specialty training in many otolaryngology diagnoses, the use of audiologists as a referral source for a telemedicine consultation would prove more efficient.

The audiologists were tasked to travel to remote areas of western Alaska and were given training on how to obtain a relevant history and perform an ENT examination.

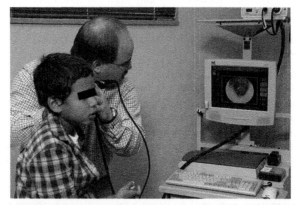

Fig. 4. An example of a patient undergoing video otoscopic imaging for a store-and-forward telemedicine encounter at the Alaska Native Medical Center. The consulting otolaryngologist can review the patient information and images at a later time from a remote location. (Image *Courtesy of* the Alaska Native Tribal Health Consortium, Anchorage (AK); with permission.)

They were given equipment including a video otoscope, a digital camera, document scanners, portable audiometer, and portable otoacoustic emissions testing units that they used to collect relevant clinical information for review by the remote otolaryngologist (**Fig. 5**). More than 94% of all the remote village visits occurred in the course of 4 to 5 days, and expenses associated with the project included salary and benefits for the audiologist as well as travel costs including airfare and lodging.[8]

A total of 1458 patients were examined by an audiologist and underwent telemedicine consultation during the course of 54 trips to remote villages in western Alaska. Twenty-seven percent of patients seen by the audiologist were considered unnecessary referrals that did not result in the generation of a telemedicine consultation.[8] This represents a significant time saving for the clinician who otherwise might see these patients in a traditional face-to-face clinic. Twenty-six percent of patients seen by the audiologist were able to have surgical intervention recommended based solely on information obtained during the course of the telemedicine consultation, which could generate potential cost savings because patients would not need to travel from remote areas for a preoperative evaluation until the day of their surgery. In summary, 67% of patients were able to have a treatment plan developed as a result of the telemedicine encounter, whereas only 15% of patients were referred to the regional ENT clinic to be seen for an in-person examination. The investigators calculated that the cost to run the program was $141,114, whereas the travel costs avoided by using telemedicine were $496,420.[8]

Previous investigators have pointed out that prolonged wait times and large patient queues lead to inefficiency, including inappropriate or wasted appointments.

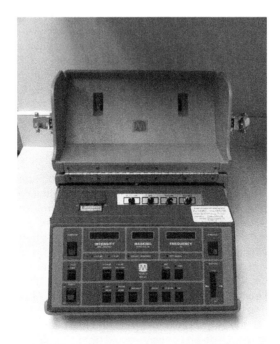

Fig. 5. A portable audiometer, which is one of the pieces of mobile equipment used by audiologists in Alaska who travel to remote villages to serve as the source for telemedicine otolaryngology consults at the Alaska Native Medical Center.

Audiologists are able to handle a large number of issues independently of a physician, and many of the patients referred to an otolaryngologist in this study likely could have been referred directly to an audiologist.[8] In a traditional practice, many of these patients would be seen in person, resulting in a potentially wasted clinic visit. Twenty-seven percent of patients were able to have surgical intervention scheduled solely from a telemedicine consultation, which is also beneficial because it spares the patient the cost of traveling to the regional medical center solely for a preoperative evaluation. Only 16% of patients required referral to the regional ENT clinic, possibly because Alaska Native Medical Center otolaryngologists are well versed in the use of telemedicine.[8] Cost savings associated with running a telemedicine practice are significant. The investigators note that the estimated savings of $355,505 are conservative, because it is difficult to calculate the savings in terms of time away from work, societal costs, and cost savings related to early diagnosis and shorter clinic wait times.[8] In addition, the investigators report that the total amount of time spent by an otolaryngologist on a typical store-and-forward telemedicine case is about 6 minutes, which means that telemedicine can increase efficiency and productivity by allowing providers to spend less time consulting and less time seeing inappropriate referrals.[8]

In 2009, Hofstetter and colleagues[11] at the University of Alaska performed a 16-year retrospective analysis of ENT specialty clinic wait times for all new patient referrals made before and after the introduction of telemedicine referrals at the medical center in 2002. The time difference between when the referral was made and when the ENT clinic appointment was scheduled was measured and compared between 2 groups. Before the introduction of telemedicine, the average wait time was 4.2 months, which declined to an average 2.5 months during the 6 years when the telemedicine program was running, representing a 40% decline in wait time with the introduction of telemedicine.[11] At the completion of their study, the average wait time was only 1.7 months, representing a wait time reduction of 50% during the 6 years when telemedicine was in use. Before the introduction of a telemedicine consult system, 35% of new patients were able to receive a new patient appointment within 3 months. After the telemedicine service was begun, more than 92% of patients were able to be seen within 3 months of making an appointment. The total number of ENT specialty appointments and the number of providers' remained the same during the length of the study period.[11]

Australian Programs

Queensland is the second largest state in Australia, with a land area of 1.7 million km^2 and an estimated population of 4 million people.[12,13] An otolaryngology service is provided at a hospital in Brisbane in the southeastern corner of Queensland, and patients living elsewhere often need to spend significant amounts of travel time to get to the hospital in Brisbane. In addition, the state subsidizes part of the travel costs for these patients, which amounts to a cost of AU$30 million a year to the state health authorities.[14] Queensland is therefore an ideal place to implement a tele-otolaryngology service, because it can potentially provide timely, expert care to a remote and rural community while potentially allowing significant cost savings for the state.

In November 2000, the Royal Children's Hospital in Queensland, Australia established a telepediatric service so that patients could be seen via videoconference rather than traveling from remote areas of Queensland to the hospital in Brisbane.[15] A call center was established so that select pediatricians throughout Queensland could contact the Royal Children's Hospital if a specialist referral was necessary. A referral coordinator at the call center handled the referral and ensured that an appropriate specialist responded to the request. Most (85%) of these consultations took place via videoconference and the rest were handled by telephone or e-mail. In 2007, Smith and colleagues[15] of the Royal Children's Hospital reviewed their telepediatric records to examine the costs of providing the telemedicine service to 2 regional hospitals in 5 years and compared these with the costs of providing traditional in-person specialist consultations. They took into consideration the costs of operating a telemedicine service, including the purchase of videoconference equipment to allow for remote nasopharyngolaryngoscopy, salaries for the coordinators and clinical staff, and tele-communications charges, and compared these with the costs involved in a traditional in-person encounter, including the costs for travel and accommodation for patients and their families (**Fig. 6**).

The investigators found that the total cost of providing a tele-otolaryngology consult service was $955,996, whereas the total cost of providing patients with traditional outpatient consultation was $1,553,264, with an average cost-per-consultation of $638 and $1036, respectively.[15] Given the fixed costs of $640,000 needed to purchase the equipment necessary to start a telemedicine practice, the investigators calculated that a threshold of 774 patients need to be seen in 5 years to make a telemedicine practice cost-effective. In this case, the workload was 1499 consultations, more than the threshold needed to make telemedicine consultation a cost-effective clinical tool. The investigators noted of the intangible savings generated by a telemedicine service that were mentioned in the Alaska studies: families need to spend less time traveling to appointments, take less time off work, have fewer inconveniences, and have lower out-of-pocket expenses than families who travel to the regional hospital.[16]

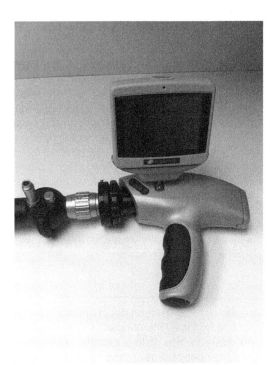

Fig. 6. A video recording system that can be directly attached to a fiberoptic scope, which allows for recording and remote viewing of a flexible fiberoptic examination.

Decision accuracy: studies in the literature

Although a significant amount of literature supports videoconferencing as a viable method of providing a teleconsultation service, there is little evidence in the literature to support the accuracy of decisions made during a telemedicine consultation. In a 2008 study, Smith and colleagues[17] studied the use of videoconferencing in place of an in-person visit with an otolaryngologist for initial assessment of children to develop a treatment plan. Specifically, they investigated whether diagnosis and management plans that were made when patients were seen via teleconference remained the same or were altered when the patients were subsequently seen by the same specialist in person. The investigators collected data on 97 patients with whom 152 tele-otolaryngology consultations were performed from 2004 to 2006. Of the original 97 patients, 75 were recommended for surgical management, whereas 19 were referred back to primary care physicians and 3 were lost to follow-up.

Patients attended a regional clinic where a videoconference was held, involving the patient and family, the referring pediatrician, and the consulting otolaryngologist.[17] A full history was obtained by the remote otolaryngologist and a comprehensive ENT examination was performed using a video otoscope remotely guided by the ENT physician. The results of diagnostic studies such as radiographs and hearing tests were also made available to the remote physician. Patients who were considered candidates for surgical management were then sent for a face-to-face consultation at the Royal Children's Hospital on the day of surgery or the day before, where they were seen by the same otolaryngologist. The otolaryngologist was unable to view the original recorded notes from the teleconference and he was tasked to review the patient information and come up with a diagnosis and treatment plan. The data from the original videoconference consultation were reviewed, compared with the data from the live patient encounter, and the diagnosis and management strategies were compared.

At the end of the study, 68 of 97 patients had undergone both a videoconference and a face-to-face encounter with an otolaryngologist.[17] The initial videoconference diagnosis was confirmed at the face-to-face encounter in 67 of 68 cases (99%). In addition, definitive surgical management correlated with the initial videoconference management plan in 63 of 68 cases (93%). Of the remaining 5 patients in whom the surgical plan differed, 4 required only minor revisions to the surgical plan, such as the inclusion or exclusion of tonsillectomy, adenoidectomy, and/or ventilation tube insertion.

The investigators concluded that their high concordance rates for diagnosis and management decisions suggest that decisions about surgical management for children assessed during teleconference are in close agreement with decisions made by the same surgeon during a face-to-face consultation. This study suggests that presurgical screening via live videoconference may be a reasonable alternative to a traditional in-person consultation, particularly in cases in which live encounters may impose a hardship on patients and their families.

Tele-otology

Telemedicine has been shown to be useful in the diagnosis and treatment of diseases involving the middle ear and tympanic membrane.[4–6] Given the success of using telemedicine in Alaska to evaluate and follow patients with otitis media, tympanic membrane perforations, tympanostomy tubes, and hearing loss, investigators recently focused their attention on determining whether store-and-forward and live videoconference telemedicine may be used to accurately plan for ear surgery.

In 2010, Kokesh and colleagues[18] at the Alaska Native Medical Center designed a study to evaluate whether telemedicine could be used in an otology practice to accurately predict the surgical procedure indicated and estimate the operative time necessary for the procedure compared with the standard in-person examination. Traditionally, patients travel to the medical center for a preoperative evaluation, at which it would be determined whether surgery was indicated. Most patients seen at Alaska Native Medical Center need to travel by air, with costs estimated between $200 and $1200 per person.[18] If patients could be evaluated for surgery and scheduled using only a telemedicine consultation, it could result in significant time and cost savings both to the patient and to the otolaryngologist.

The investigators performed a retrospective chart review to evaluate 45 cases in which major ear surgery was scheduled and performed after a telemedicine encounter, and matched these with a control group of 45 cases in which major ear surgery was performed after a traditional in-person encounter. The surgeries included in the analysis included tympanoplasty, mastoidectomy, stapes surgery, and myringoplasty. The telemedicine cases that were examined originated from providers throughout rural Alaska and were reviewed by an otolaryngologist who developed a treatment plan and confirmed the planned surgical procedure and time. All the patients were seen for a standard preoperative evaluation the day before surgery at the medical center where the history was confirmed and they underwent examination with a binocular operating microscope.

The investigators found that the surgical procedure matched the planned procedure in 40 of 45 patients (89%) in the telemedicine group and 38 of 45 patients (84%) seen during in-person consultations, with the most common change being the addition or cancellation of a canalplasty from a scheduled tympanoplasty. The time required for the planned surgery was within 30 minutes of the time scheduled for 60% of the patients evaluated by telemedicine and 62% of the patients evaluated in person, with the remained taking longer or shorter than initially planned. There was no statistically significant difference between the 2 groups.

The investigators concluded that their study supported the practice of using telemedicine to evaluate patients before surgery to avoid the cost and time associated with traveling from a remote area to see a specialist.[18] Compared with patients who were seen in person in the clinic, patient consultations held via telemedicine led to accurate surgical scheduling and time estimates. The investigators found a major benefit of telemedicine to be that it allows the otolaryngologist to directly schedule patients for surgery where appropriate, thus avoiding an unnecessary and expensive visit to the clinic. Telemedicine also allows patients to be seen in the office for an additional appointment, if necessary, to obtain a more detailed history.

In 2010, Arriaga and colleagues[19] reported their experience in developing a telemedicine-assisted neurotology service in post-Katrina Louisiana. After hurricane Katrina, the Louisiana State University Health Science Center in New Orleans had no neurotology service available. Starting in 2007, the investigators developed a telemedicine neurotology service at a clinic in Baton Rouge (LA) using a combination of real-time patient evaluation and store-and-forward telemedicine. Patients visited the clinic in Baton Rouge and a physician interacted with the patient and reviewed all the clinically relevant materials from a remote location. Baton Rouge had a full-time audiologist, nurse practitioner, and on-site neurosurgery and otolaryngology services. A neurotologist was available on site only 3 days a month for in-person examinations and for surgery. The rest of the time was spent at a hospital in Pittsburgh.

During 12 months of operation, the investigators reported that there were a total of 450 telemedicine patient encounters, 800 on-site patient visits, and 150 operative procedures including 24 neurotologic skull base procedures. Of the patients undergoing surgery, 24% were seen for the first time in person by the neurotologist on the day of surgery. The investigators concluded that their successful experience validates the role of telemedicine in preoperative planning, particularly in a setting in which resources may be limited, patients may live in isolated areas, or in areas where otolaryngologists are in short supply.[19]

The investigators of this study held direct discussions with third-party payers to ensure that there were opportunities for reimbursement, and they were able to obtain explicit written approval from private insurers for physician reimbursement using standard management codes. The issue of reimbursement continues to represent a major barrier to wider acceptance and use of telemedicine in otolaryngology, and the success of the investigators in negotiating a reimbursement schedule with private insurers is encouraging for the future.

An article published in 2008 by Shapiro and colleagues[20] of New York University dealt with the issue of using telemedicine to perform remote intraoperative testing and monitoring of cochlear implant devices during implantation surgery. The investigators stated that intraoperative testing of cochlear implant devices has been routinely performed in their institution for the last 2 decades to provide immediate feedback to the implant team to confirm the integrity of the device.[20] For example, intraoperative impedance measurements may indicate whether the electrode array is faulty and allow the surgeon to replace the malfunctioning device while the patient is still in the operating suite and under anesthesia. Some of the information obtained during testing includes impedance telemetry, electrically evoked stapedial reflex threshold, and neural response telemetry. This testing was traditionally performed by an audiologist who physically traveled to the operating room (OR); however, this requires a significant time and cost commitment, because there is typically minimal to no payment for these services. The investigators believed that the ability to remotely monitor and test cochlear implant devices during implantation surgery would improve both time and cost efficiency for both the audiologist and the surgeon involved.[20]

Software from the Cochlear Corporation and Advanced Bionics Corporation was configured by the investigators to perform remote testing of cochlear implants. The investigators subsequently took a series of 8 patients, 4 of whom underwent traditional in-person testing of the cochlear implant during surgery and 4 of whom underwent remote testing. The investigators measured the amount of time required for each mode of testing and compared the two. They found that the average time required for remote testing was 7.5 minutes, with an average of 9 minutes spent by the audiologist. The average time required for in-person monitoring was 15 minutes, and the average amount of time spent by the audiologist was a total of 93 minutes.

The discrepancy between remote and in-person monitoring is largely caused by the amount of time required for the audiologist to arrive in the OR, the amount of time spent by the audiologist waiting in the OR for the surgeon to be ready, and the amount of time spent walking back from the OR to the main audiology offices.[20] The time required for the monitoring was similar between the 2 groups. New York University typically performs approximately 170 cochlear implants per year, the investigators calculated that the difference between 9 minutes for remote testing and 96 minutes for in-person testing equates to a total difference of 238 hours for the year in lost time for their audiologist, which is a total of 6.35 weeks of lost productivity using traditional in-person implant monitoring compared with remote monitoring. The investigators conclude that remote intraoperative monitoring during cochlear implant surgery is feasible, timesaving, practical, and efficient.[20]

TELEMEDICINE AND SPEECH AND LANGUAGE DISORDERS

Approximately 14 million individuals in the United States have a speech, voice, or language disorder.[21] Proper diagnosis and treatment are key to ensuring that an individual has full learning and employment opportunities, but the availability and accessibility of care is a significant problem for people who live in remote areas of the United States.[22] The diagnosis of speech and language disorders traditionally requires a face-to-face encounter between a patient and a clinician. The factors related to the diagnosis of a speech and language disorder are based on language use, auditory perceptual features of speech, and visual characteristics of speech movements. Because many of these features are amenable to interpretation at a distance, there is a potential role for the use of telemedicine in diagnosing speech and language disorders.

Using telemedicine in speech and language pathology was first pioneered more than a decade ago at the Mayo Clinic with the assistance of satellites launched by the National Aeronautics and Space Administration. In 1997, Duffy and colleagues[23] had 8 patients undergo remote speech and language assessment using 24 separate videotaped samples, with a second clinician present on site to assess the reliability of the remote observer's assessments. They then compared the diagnosis and looked for agreement between the remote observe and the in-person clinician.

The investigators found that the concordance between the remote observer and the in-person clinician was 96%. They found that all of their patients were satisfied with the remote encounter. The investigators concluded that speech pathology remote consultations can contribute to medical diagnosis and management of numerous communication disorders, particularly in patients who do not have access to services locally.[23]

A study in 2003 from Tripler Army Medical Center further details the use of telemedicine in providing voice therapy to patients.[24] Seventy-two patients were seen in the Tripler Army Medical Center Speech Pathology Clinic with a variety of disorders, including vocal nodules, vocal fold edema, and vocal fold paralysis, and were randomly assigned to participate in one of 2 groups. The first group was conventional voice therapy, with the patient and clinician in the same room, and the second group was remote voice therapy, with the patient and clinician in adjacent rooms interacting via a real-time videoconference. The investigators examined voice quality as assessed independently by 2 speech-language pathologists independently, performed acoustic analysis, and assessed patient satisfaction. The investigators found that both the conventional therapy and remote therapy groups showed statistically significant improvement in their voices as indicated by the factors discussed earlier. Although both groups improved significantly after receiving therapy, there was no significant difference between the conventional and remote voice therapy groups in any of the factors mentioned earlier. The investigators concluded that voice therapy delivered remotely is as effective as traditional in-person voice therapy, and that it may be a valuable tool in treating patients who live in geographically remote areas, who suffer from physical difficulties that make it difficult to travel, or for patients who need to relocate and who would otherwise need to seek a new provider.[24]

In 2008, Lewis and colleagues[24] from the University of Sydney and the University of Queensland in Australia published a study comparing the use of traditional live delivery of the Lidcombe Program for Early Stuttering Intervention with a group who underwent the same program remotely. They noted that regular speech-language services are not available to 30% of the nation's population who live in remote and rural areas, and that most rural Australian towns do not receive a local speech-language pathology service. Therefore, an investigation into the use of telemedicine to deliver these services could potentially be significant. They developed a blinded, randomized controlled trial in which 22 school-aged children with stuttering were randomly assigned to either the control group, which underwent the standard Lidcombe program, or to the experimental group, which underwent a remote telemedicine version of the Lidcombe program. The primary outcome of the study was the percentage of syllables stuttered in each group, and the secondary outcomes included treatment time and patient satisfaction.

At the outset of the study the percentages of syllables stuttered in the control group and experimental groups were 4.5% and 6.7%, respectively. After 9 months of treatment with the Lidcombe program, the percentage of syllables stuttered decreased from 4.5% to 1.9% in the control group and from 6.7% to 1.1% in the experimental group, representing a statistically significant improvement in stuttering of 69% in the experimental group compared with the control group. The caveat is that it took patients in the telemedicine group an average of 62.9 weeks to complete stage 1 of the Lidcombe program compared with an average of 26.9 weeks in the control group. The investigators concluded that the evidence suggests that telehealth delivery of the Lidcombe Program is an effective means of treating stuttering in children. Although telemedicine delivery of the Lidcombe is not presently as cost-efficient as traditional in-person therapy, it remains a useful tool for providing access to speech-language pathology services to children and families who live in rural and remote locations.

SUMMARY

Telemedicine has the potential to change the way that health care is delivered in the United States and across the world. Perhaps the most promising aspect of telemedicine is its ability to bring health care services to patients living in remote and isolated areas who otherwise might not have access to specialty medical care. In addition, telemedicine has the potential to provide significant time and cost savings for medical providers.

The telemedicine programs at the Alaska Native Medical Center and at the Royal Children's Hospital in Queensland, Australia, have been successful, and have helped to improve the delivery of subspecialty surgical care to patients living in isolated areas, as well as generating significant cost and time savings, both for patients and for the otolaryngology practices. The development of a remote telemedical neurotology service deployed in post-Katrina Louisiana shows another potential use of telemedicine in extending health care to those living in areas affected by large-scale disasters.

Although there clearly is a role for telemedicine in otolaryngology, significant issues remain before wider acceptance can occur. For example, the issue of reimbursement from private insurers and the government represents a significant barrier to greater adoption of telemedicine technology. In addition, although various investigators have shown that a telemedicine practice has the potential to generate significant cost savings, the start-up costs involved in a creating a telemedicine practice can also be significant. In addition, although the initial evidence is promising, more work remains to be done to ensure that telemedicine is an accurate and effective means for developing a diagnosis and treatment plan. Regardless of the challenges, the future of telemedicine continues to be promising because of its capability to fulfill a specific health care need. As technology continues to become cheaper and more widely available, there will likely be a larger role for telemedicine in the future.

REFERENCES

1. Sclafani AP, Heneghan C, Ginsburg J, et al. Teleconsultation in otolaryngology: live versus store and forward consultations. Otolaryngol Head Neck Surg 1999; 120:62–72.

2. Bondy J, Berman S, Glander J, et al. Direct expenditures related to otitis media diagnosis: extrapolations from a pediatric Medicaid cohort. Pediatrics 2000; 105:E72.
3. Patricoski C, Kokesh J, Ferguson AS, et al. A comparison of in-person examination and video otoscope imaging for tympanostomy tube follow-up. Telemed J E Health 2003;9:331–43.
4. Aronzon A, Ross T, Kazahaya K, et al. Diagnosis of middle ear disease using tympanograms and digital imaging. Otolaryngol Head Neck Surg 2004;131: 917–20.
5. Lundberg T, Westman G, Hellstrom S, et al. Digital imaging and telemedicine as a tool for studying inflammatory conditions in the middle ear – evaluation of image quality and agreement between examiners. Int J Pediatr Otorhinolaryngol 2008; 72:73–9.
6. Kokesh J, Ferguson AS, Patricoski C, et al. Digital images for postsurgical follow-up of tympanostomy tubes in remote Alaska. Otolaryngol Head Neck Surg 2008; 139:87–93.
7. US Census Bureau. Statistical analysis of the United States. Atlanta (GA): US Departtment of Commerce; 2000.
8. Kokesh J, Ferguson AS, Patricoski C, et al. Traveling an audiologist to provide otolaryngology care using store-and-forward telemedicine. Telemed J E Health 2009;15:758–63.
9. Alaska Center for Rural Health. Alaska's allied health workforce: a statewide assessment. Anchorage (AK): University of Anchorage; 2001.
10. Smart DR, Sellers J. Physician characteristics and distribution: 2008 edition. Chicago: American Medical Association; 2008.
11. Hofstetter PJ, Kokesh J, Ferguson AS, et al. The impact of telehealth on wait time for ENT specialty care. Telemed J E Health 2009;16:551–6.
12. Department of Foreign Affairs and Trade: Queensland facts [online]. Brisbane (Australia) 1995. Available at: http://www.about-australia.com/facts/queensland. Accessed August 28th, 2010.
13. Australian Bureau of Statistics: Australian Demographic Statistics, catalogue number 3101.0 [online]. Brisbane (Australia). Available at: http://www.abs.gov. au/ausstats/abs@.nsf/mf/3101.0. Accessed August 28th, 2010.
14. Queensland Health. Queensland Health annual report 2002-2003. Brisbane (Australia): Queensland Government; 2003. p. 1–93.
15. Smith AC, Schuffman P, Wootton R. The costs and potential savings of a novel telepaediatric service in Queensland. BMC Health Serv Res 2007;7:35.
16. Smith AC, Youngberry K, Isles A, et al. The family costs of attending hospital outpatient appointments via videoconference and in person. Telemed J E Health 2003;9:58–61.
17. Smith AC, Dowthwaite S, Agnew J, et al. Concordance between real-time telemedicine assessments and face-to-face consultations in paediatric otolaryngology. Med J Aust 2008;188:457–60.
18. Kokesh J, Ferguson AS, Patricoski C. Preoperative planning for ear surgery using store-and-forward telemedicine. Otolaryngol Head Neck Surg 2010;143:253–7.
19. Arriaga MA, Nuss D, Scrantz K, et al. Telemedicine-assisted neurotology in post-Katrina southeast Louisiana. Otol Neurotol 2010;31:524–7.
20. Shapiro WH, Huang T, Shaw T, et al. Remote intraoperative monitoring during cochlear implant surgery is feasible and efficient. Otol Neurotol 2008;29:495–8.
21. Research in human communication. Bethesda (MD): National Institute on Deafness and Other Communication Disorders; 1995.

22. Mashima PA, Birkmire-Peters DP, Syms MJ, et al. Telehealth: voice therapy using telecommunications technology. Am J Speech Lang Pathol 2003;12:432–9.

23. Duffy JR, Werven GW, Aronson AE. Telemedicine and the diagnosis of speech and language disorders. Mayo Clin Proc 1997;72:1116–22.

24. Lewis C, Packman A, Onslow M, et al. A phase II trial of telehealth delivery of the Lidcombe program of early stuttering intervention. Am J Speech Lang Pathol 2008;17:139–49.

Successful Models for Telehealth

Elizabeth A. Krupinski, PhD[a],*, Tim Patterson, BA[b,c,d],
Cameron D. Norman, PhD[c,e], Yehudah Roth, MD[c,e,f,g],
Ziad ElNasser, MD, PhD[c,e,h], Ziad Abdeen, PhD[c,d,e],
Arnold Noyek, MD, FRCSC[c,d,e,g,i,j], Abi Sriharan, MSc[g],
Andrew Ignatieff, BA[c,g], Sandra Black, MD, FRCPC[k],
Morris Freedman, MD, FRCPC[l]

KEYWORDS

• Telehealth • Telemedicine • Sustainability • Models

Successful telemedicine programs that went beyond demonstration and pilot project efforts started appearing in the United States in the late 1980s and early 1990s,[1,2] and many of them are still providing valuable services to a variety of patient populations. In the early days of telemedicine, the focus was mainly on providing services to rural or remote populations, and environments with special needs such as prison populations.

[a] Department of Radiology, University of Arizona, 1609 North Warren Building 211, Tucson, AZ 85724, USA
[b] Department of Telehealth, Baycrest, 3560 Bathurst Street, Toronto, Canada M6A 2E1
[c] Canada International Scientific Exchange Program, 700 University Avenue, Suite 8600, Toronto, Canada M5G 1×6
[d] Health Research Institute, Al Quds University, Jerusalem Beit Hanina, PO Box 51000, West Bank
[e] Department of Public Health Sciences, University of Toronto, 155 College Street, Toronto, Canada M5T 3M7
[f] Department of Otolaryngology–Head & Neck Surgery, Edith Wolfson Medical Center, Tel Aviv University Sackler School Faculty of Medicine, 62 HaLohamim Street, PO Box 5, Holon 58100, Israel
[g] The Peter A. Silverman Centre for International Health, Mount Sinai Hospital, 600 University Avenue, Toronto, Canada M5G 1×5
[h] Department of Medicine, King Abdulla University Hospital, Jordan University of Science and Technology, PO Box 360001, Irbid 22110, Jordan
[i] Department of Otolaryngology/Head and Neck Surgery, University of Toronto, 190 Elizabeth Street, RFE Building, Toronto, Canada M5G 2N2
[j] International Continuing Education, University of Toronto, Faculty of Medicine, 500 University Avenue, Suite 650, Toronto, Canada M5G 1V7
[k] Division of Neurology, Department of Medicine, Sunnybrook Health Sciences Centre, Rotman Research Institute, University of Toronto, 399 Bathurst Street, Toronto, Canada M5T 2S8
[l] Division of Neurology, Department of Medicine, Mt Sinai Hospital, Rotman Research Institute, Baycrest, University and Health Network, University of Toronto, 3560 Bathurst Street, Toronto, Canada M6A 2E1
* Corresponding author.
E-mail address: krupinski@radiology.arizona.edu

Otolaryngol Clin N Am 44 (2011) 1275–1288
doi:10.1016/j.otc.2011.08.004
0030-6665/11/$ – see front matter © 2011 Elsevier Inc. All rights reserved.

Key Points: SUCCESSFUL TELEHEALTH MODELS

- Telehealth facilitates continuing professional development and knowledge exchange across large distances and in hard-to-access locations, and is ideal for targeting international audiences and allowing health care professionals to share knowledge face to face without constraints of geography.
- Planning and maintaining a successful a telemedicine program is challenging, and there are often barriers to developing sustainable telehealth programs.
- The key to success of any telemedicine program is training and education.
- Evaluation is core to the success of any telemedicine program—not only understanding benefits and limitations of technology, but how components work together as a whole system in conjunction with the user.
- There is no single business model that will work for every program, but there are models for analyzing the costs and benefits of conducting telemedicine that are useful.

Today telemedicine is much more far reaching and there has been substantial growth in areas such as urban, school, occupational, first-responder, and home telemedicine activities. It is impossible to review all of the successful telemedicine activities occurring today because they are extensive and varied. Instead, the authors present brief summaries of two very successful telemedicine programs that can serve as models for those interested in developing a new program or those with existing programs looking for ways to improve sustainability and increase their outreach.

When establishing a successful telemedicine program, it is important and useful to consider what others have accomplished and what precedents have been set. In particular, there have been significant efforts in recent years to establish standards and guidelines for telemedicine practices. Some of these are more technical in nature, describing the type of equipment that should be used and what the minimum performance standards are, whereas others are practice guidelines detailing how specific types of evaluations and examinations should be conducted in the telemedicine environment. For example, radiology has several technical and practice guidelines in place for digital image acquisition, storage, transfer, and display via Picture Archiving and Communications Systems (PACS) and teleradiology[3–5]; and the Society of American Gastrointestinal and Endoscopic Surgeons has guidelines for the surgical practice of telemedicine.[6] The American Telemedicine Association has made significant progress in establishing both general guidelines for the practice of telemedicine[7] and practice guidelines for specific clinical specialties.[8–11] Although to date there are no established practice guidelines for teleotolaryngology, there have been some successful projects that can serve as practice models.[12–14]

THE ARIZONA TELEMEDICINE PROGRAM

The Arizona Telemedicine Program (ATP), funded by state funding and grants, was established in May 1997 to enhance health care delivery to medically underserved populations throughout the state using telemedicine technologies. The program was founded on 8 core policies,[15] key of which were:

- Creation of a single state-wide multiservice telemedicine program
- Provide access to the program's telecommunications infrastructure for all legitimate health care organizations in the state

- Encourage the development of interoperability of all telemedicine facilities
- Develop an open staff model for participation of physicians as service providers for multiple health care organizations
- Promote best practice guidelines that are evidence-based and supported by clinical research
- Operate the program as a virtual organization that would be inclusive and create incentives for all health care organizations to participate in a state-wide single telemedicine program.

At its formation, the founders of the program recognized that to be successful it would have to do more than simply offer teleconsultation services; the program would have to be a comprehensive entity that provided infrastructure, clinical services, training, and professional education (**Fig. 1**). In terms of infrastructure, the ATP operates a private broad-band telecommunications network, the Arizona Telemedicine Network (ATN), which links more than 170 sites in more than 70 communities across the state. The network serves as an umbrella organization for 55 independent health care organizations located in such diverse settings as academic hospitals, community health centers, Indian Health Service facilities, the Department of Corrections, schools, and even patient's homes.

Telehealth services have been offered in more than 60 clinical subspecialties, with teleradiology serving as the core service to approximately 25 hospitals and having conducted more than 1 million primary reads! The other subspecialties use both real-time videoconferencing (VTC) and store-and-forward technologies; at the hub site alone more than 15,000 teleconsultations have been conducted, with telepsychiatry as the main real-time application and teledermatology as the main store-and-forward application. In addition, more than 25,000 teleconsults have been conducted in the Department of Corrections since 1997, and it is estimated that 80% of the specialty consultations for the Arizona Department of Corrections are delivered directly into the prisons by telemedicine, thus avoiding tens of thousands of miles of travel by guarded prisoners every year. As an open service model, the ATN also connects non-ATP telehealth networks throughout the state; this includes several affiliated telepsychiatry networks in Arizona that have conducted more than 50,000 telepsychiatry patient sessions to date.

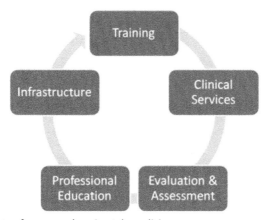

Fig. 1. Components of a comprehensive telemedicine program.

The key to success of any telemedicine program is training and education.[16] Although telemedicine is really just another mode of health care delivery, there are some very unique aspects to it that must be considered. For example, not only must the users have some basic technological skills to effectively use the specialized equipment used in telemedicine (**Fig. 2**), they also need to understand the limitations and benefits of those new technologies in terms of providing clinical information to the relevant users who need to render diagnostic decisions based on the data provided by those technologies. There are also "social" issues of which users need to be aware: how does one establish rapport with a patient over video, where should one look during a VTC consult to make eye contact (at the camera or at the monitor?), and do different cultures view teleservices differently (eg, Native Americans)? In addition, the authors have found that in many rural sites the turnover in health care personnel is very high, affecting the consistency with which services can be offered.[17]

Training Programs for Telehealth Services

To combat this problem, the ATP offers bimonthly training programs with two options. The first provides an overview of telemedicine, covering everything from business aspects to technology. The second focuses on clinical applications. Both provide hands-on opportunities for participants to interact and use various telemedicine technologies and equipment. The training is free to individuals associated with Arizona programs and charges a nominal fee to out-of-state and international participants, contributing to the sustainability of the program overall. To maintain the lessons learned in these training sessions, the ATP also offers on-site follow-up training once a site acquires and installs its equipment, so that the users can familiarize themselves with the technology in the environment in which it will be used. Users are encouraged to renew their training on a regular basis to not only refresh their basic skills, but also to keep abreast of any changes in technology and practice standards and guidelines.

The ATP also provides approximately 500 hours annually of interactive continuing medical education and continuing education to participants in remote locations in Arizona and New Mexico using bidirectional video. Participants, who would normally be required to take costly trips, spending valuable time away from their practices to meet

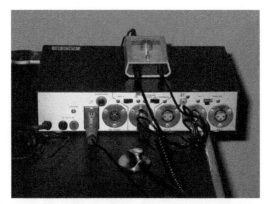

Fig. 2. A electronic stethoscope. Most health care providers new to telemedicine will not be familiar with the electronic stethoscope in terms of its operation or subtle differences compared with the traditional stethoscope, so hands-on training sessions include familiarization with these types of specialized technologies.

their annual educational requirements for licensure, are able to meet or exceed their requirement by participating in grand rounds from their own location, at their convenience, free of charge. Offerings across the network over the years have included grand rounds in ATP Clinical Care, Medicine, Psychiatry, Nursing, Geriatrics, Surgery, OBGYN, Pediatrics, Integrative Medicine, Public Health, Arizona Public Health Preparedness, and Informatics (**Fig. 3**). Although these offerings do not provide income to the program, they do "advertise" the capabilities of telemedicine and the ATP to health care providers across the state, and often this is the first introduction to telemedicine that many providers have.

Evaluation of Telehealth Programs

Evaluation is key to the success of any telemedicine program.[18] Not only is it important to understand the benefits and limitations of the individual pieces of technology to be used in telehealth consultations, but it is important also to understand how the various components work together as a whole system. One factor that many evaluations fail to take into account when doing evaluations in telemedicine is the user. Human factors in telemedicine applications are increasingly being recognized as an important evaluation parameter, but it is still a relatively forgotten component of the telemedicine encounter.[19]

Aside from evaluating the technology and general practice of telemedicine, it is important for a successful program to assess itself on a periodic basis. There are no set methods to carry out such evaluations, but tools exist that can be modified or adapted to particular situations.[20,21] Some of the basic information that can be tracked to assess program progress includes number of consults per month, number of real-time versus store-and-forward consults, referring and consulting sites, referring and consulting clinicians, case subspecialty, patient demographics (age, gender, major complaint), primary diagnosis, and primary recommendation. These key

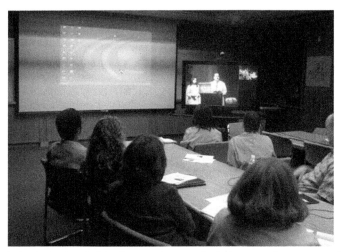

Fig. 3. Typical continuing education session conducted remotely over a telemedicine network. The audience is in the foreground and the guest lecturer (from Panama in this case) is seen on the monitor at the back. The lecture material can be displayed through a separate channel on the screen to the left of the video monitor for simultaneous viewing of the material and the speakers.

variables can be tracked and over time can provide a global picture about the status of a program, changes in case types and case loads, types of services being requested, and so forth.[17,22,23] Keeping track of this type of information helps with program sustainability in the sense that it allows for better and more efficient staffing as well as more efficient use of services and personnel, and allows a program to make changes if significant trends in service loads and specialties are observed.

Skills of Telemedicine Staff

One of the challenges in sustaining a telemedicine program is not only having a core champion to promote the concept, but having the right people to support that concept and make the everyday running of the program efficient and effective. One of the ways to succeed in this is to have a set of established job descriptions for the key personnel of the program. For example, the job description for an ATP Rural Site Coordinator specifies that he or she must have experience of working in a medical practice environment including patient scheduling, and must have the ability to establish priorities according to preestablished policies and guidelines. The Coordinator also must possess good interpersonal skills and be comfortable in patient care settings, understanding the implications of patient confidentiality and privacy issues. He or she must have strong organizational skills and the ability to work with other health care providers, and have strong data-handling abilities. His or her responsibilities include: operating and maintaining telemedicine equipment; assisting the rural practitioner during the consult; collecting necessary transaction data including patient demographics and record information; participating in user group forums; collaborating in the development of protocols; overseeing integration of rotating medical students and residents in teleconsultation sessions; and working with the Evaluator to collect relevant assessment data. In addition, each job description indicates the chain of responsibility and who each person reports to.

Business and Operational Models for Telemedicine

The final key to success and sustainability of any telemedicine program is its business model. There is no single business model that will work for every program because every program offers different services, operates in different environments, and is reliant on different amounts of external funding (eg, grants). There are, however, several publications detailing several business models and/or analyzing the costs and benefits of conducting telemedicine.[24–27] The ATP has developed a virtual organization connecting organizations throughout the state of Arizona. It uses a membership formalized through legal contracts in a shared-cost model to capitalize on economies of scale (an application services model or ASP) by sharing services at lower costs. Sharing services across multiple health care organizations can contribute to success and sustainability. **Fig. 4** shows the basic components of the ATP ASP business model.

In **Fig. 4**, each layer supports the layer(s) on top of it. The vendor services layer represents the physical infrastructure of the network (eg, leased T-1 and T-3 telecommunications lines). The infrastructure layer contains the actual telecommunications infrastructure once installed. This layer represents services that support the basic ATP structure including telecommunications, marketing services, funding support, and grant writing. It is the foundation of the program and is the core of what all clients obtain when they become a member. The operational services layer includes the daily operations: clinic operations, equipment installation, practice management, training, transcription, billing, and reimbursement.

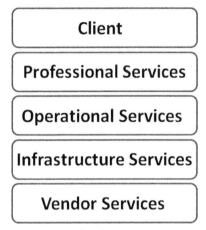

Fig. 4. The membership/business model for the Arizona Telemedicine Program.

The operational services level includes actual services supported by or supplied by the program, including health care provider services, clinical protocol development, continuing education, quality assurance and quality control, credentialing, licensing, and legal. Finally comes the client layer; clients can be patients, payers, or businesses that use the various services supported by the program. Once members, the clients can choose (and pay for) those services they want. For example, an organization may choose to use the clinical services for teleconsultations but may have no need for distance education services, so they pay only for one and not the other. In this way the model is very flexible and clients need to purchase only those services in which they are interested. It also allows clients to maintain their traditional patient referral patterns. Clients may choose to purchase, for example, access to the telecommunications infrastructure but not the clinical services operated by the ATP hub site. Instead, with the telecommunications link they can connect to their existing specialty-referring site if it is on the network. Thus, the ATP model is referred to as an open network whereby individual sites can connect with each other rather than with a central hub facility only. This membership-based ASP business model has provided a steady revenue stream for the program which, when combined with revenue from clinical services reimbursement and external funding for equipment upgrades and special projects, has contributed to the sustainability of the program for nearly 15 years.

BAYCREST TELEHEALTH PROGRAM

Health care is a common language of need that transcends culture, religion, and nationality, and is vital to the advancement of any society. One of the limiting factors influencing health care delivery worldwide, but particularly in the developing world, is the availability of skilled professionals to serve society in meeting its health needs and goals. Telehealth, a developing medium that facilitates continuing professional development and knowledge exchange across large distances and in hard-to-access locations,[28] is ideal for targeting international audiences and allowing health care professionals to share knowledge face to face without constraints of geography.

Accordingly, the Peter A. Silverman Global eHealth Program (PASGeP) was established in 2005 to create an international telehealth network with Canadian, Israeli,

Jordanian, and Palestinian sites. A major goal was to help build bridges to peace in the Middle East through health care initiatives, building on the pioneering work of the Canada International Scientific Exchange Program (CISEPO) and its accomplishments over the past 2 decades.[29,30]

The PASGeP was launched with the signing of a Memorandum of Understanding among Baycrest, CISEPO, the Department of Public Health Sciences at the University of Toronto, and the Peter A. Silverman Center for International Health, Mount Sinai Hospital. The program was designed to test and evaluate a telehealth-based continuing education program for use in promotion of cooperation and knowledge exchange within the network of regions in partnership with CISEPO. Since 1995, CISEPO has brought together Israelis, Jordanians, and Palestinians around the common goal of enhancing health and promoting cooperative dialog.[30,31] Its activities range from numerous continuing education events, to subspecialty surgery, to community hearing screening centers that have assessed hundreds of thousands of infants.[31] The CISEPO partnerships involve a 3-part approach to partnership development anchored by health care service, research, and policy-related health promotion.

For the pilot project, each Canadian and Middle East site installed telehealth equipment suited to their local needs and capabilities. Baycrest, which serves as the hub, received additional television equipment to allow for broadcast-quality production capabilities, and assumed the production and coordination responsibilities. The telecasts have emphasized a series of programs involving a core collaboration of Canadian, Israeli, Jordanian, and Palestinian sites using "on the ground" infrastructure and relationships, and established relationships within the CISEPO network. Regional hospitals equipped with videoconferencing equipment outside the collaboration covered by the Memorandum of Understanding also participate in the programming. The University of Toronto City-Wide Behavioral Neurology Rounds, Co-Chaired by Dr Morris Freedman and Dr Sandra Black, were selected as the series for the international program. The Behavioral Neurology Rounds are broadcast weekly to Toronto sites using the Ontario Telemedicine Network (OTN), while the international broadcasts occur once per month during the academic year.

The cross-border programming is designed for academic continuing professional development, international relationship building toward cooperation, and demonstrating the power of health care as a common language to bring people together. The PASGeP has appointed telehealth directors to plan the content and oversee local coordination of the series. The directors for the Middle East are also the 3 CISEPO Program Directors: Dr Yehudah Roth (Israeli program), Dr Ziad ElNasser (Jordanian program), and Dr Ziad Abdeen (Palestinian program). For Canada, the telehealth initiative is coordinated by Dr Morris Freedman, Tim Patterson, and Andrew Ignatieff.

Programming

The telecasts are accredited as a group learning activity as defined by The Maintenance of Certification Program of The Royal College of Physicians and Surgeons of Canada. This accreditation, while being relevant for Canadian participation in the program, is also important to the international audience as a means of enhancing the credibility of content. In addition to seeking accreditation, the programming aimed to implement television-quality production levels to make the telecasts more seamless. The rationale for such emphasis on production quality was that technical/production problems or lack of preparedness detract from the audience's engagement with the content and medium.

The topical focus of the telecasts is centered on neurobehavioral impairment including exploration of issues pertaining to Alzheimer disease, frontotemporal dementia, and cognitive impairment due to Parkinson disease. Programming typically involves case presentations with live participation from either patient and/or family in person or via telecast. This approach enables the telecast audience to interact with the audience and provide feedback to the attending physicians about possible diagnoses and treatment prospects. Remote sites are not allowed to videotape the programming, due to patient confidentiality. Fostering interaction, rather than providing simple didactic instruction, is an essential component of building relationships between the sites and enhancing the format's knowledge transfer potential. Anecdotally, the rounds' participants have commented that the patient presentations focus their attention and empathy on the common humanitarian aspects of the case—the diagnostic and management challenges and the need to alleviate suffering in each patient and family. This focus seems to suspend geographic and political barriers, as the attendees collaboratively solve problems and learn together.

A program script is prepared for each telecast, allowing all sites to be aware of the flow of the program so that they can be prepared for the interactive discussion periods; this was viewed very positively by program coordinators at each site. The Chair of the series, based at Baycrest, has responsibility for coordinating the content for the international program. This role has served as a platform for promoting learning and teaching on the art and science of providing education through the telehealth medium. Some pivotal lessons include learning about where to stand in relation to camera positions, awareness of camera angles, and methods to invoke and provoke discussion from the remote sites to encourage interaction.

Production

Baycrest television production capabilities were upgraded through the PASGeP initiative to include:

1. Two-camera shoot with the ability for multiple camera shots
2. A monitor for the Chair and presenter to see the remote sites and maintain eye contact with participants at these sites
3. Microphones in the ceiling so that the Baycrest audience (local) can conduct a dialog with the presenter without having to repeat the question to the remote audiences
4. Constant monitoring of the bridge (described below) to allow for the intricacies of health care programming.

This equipment made for a strong production base of operations that could accommodate large local audiences and deliver a quality program.

Resolve Collaboration Services was hired to accomplish the international bridging, and OTN bridged the Toronto, Ontario sites. Bridging services allow for multisite interaction. These technical capabilities facilitate a smoother production that allows the audiences to concentrate on the content rather than on the production inadequacies.

Monitoring and Evaluation Framework

A framework and methodology for evaluating the impact of international telehealth programming was developed to guide the evaluation and monitoring activities. The first step in this process was the development of a program logic model, which maps out the inputs, activities, and expected outputs, and planned outcomes associated with the goals of PASGeP. The logic model outlined the purpose and scope of the program in simple terms, and was used to frame the evaluation and monitoring efforts and to assist in program communications (**Fig. 5**).

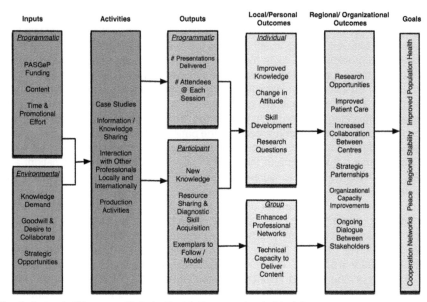

Fig. 5. Peter A. Silverman Global eHealth Program Logic Model.

Guiding Research Questions

The program evaluation was designed to explore the feasibility of using telehealth to provide knowledge exchange opportunities between health professionals in the Middle East and Canada, and the level of satisfaction with the programming in terms of quality and appropriateness. A secondary aim was to serve as a means of formulating research questions to guide the development of the program beyond its pilot phase.

Monitoring and evaluation activities consisted of observational notes recorded at each international event, including documenting attendance from each site, a timed log of events corresponding to significant moments for each telecast (eg, start time, transmission difficulties, questions, and discussion), and a synopsis of the interactions and discussions that took place during the program in terms of audience participation.

The initial evaluation activities have focused on determining the extent to which the PASGeP format was consistent with the needs of the program participants and institutions at each site. Individual, in-depth interviews were conducted in person or via telephone with the site leaders at each of the 3 main Middle East sites, and with the production leader and series Chair at Baycrest, to explore the degree to which PASGeP was addressing the local professional needs, expectations, and providing quality educational opportunities for participants at each site in the first year. The interviews also identified areas for further study and programming modification. The results of the needs assessment were then presented to the CISEPO and PASGeP leadership team and were incorporated into planning actions for the second year at a meeting of all program leads held via videoconference.

In Year Two, the series evolved from an exclusive Canadian programming and production focus to include the Middle East sites hosting telecasts. This expansion gave the Middle East sites an equal opportunity to share their knowledge and created a sense of ownership within the international network. A second round of interviews was conducted with the regional coordinators in Year Two to discuss progress and further issues for programming as a means of program monitoring and ongoing needs assessments.

Summary Results

The results from both sets of interviews suggested that:

1. The production quality and transmission was consistently good
2. Participants had a high level of satisfaction with the quality of the speakers and the expertise made available through the programming
3. The strategy used to encourage and respond to questions was effective, but consistent dialog between the sites was not being fully realized
4. Overall satisfaction with the program was high; participant leaders believed the program provided considerable value-added benefits to their work and organizations, while supporting positive relationships within and between the regions. PAS-GeP was viewed as opening up new collaborative and learning opportunities with others both within the hospital and in different departments within the regions
5. The general style of the programming and the length (60–75 minutes) were agreed as being ideal for learning and maintaining focus. Programming was perceived to be at its best when: (1) patients were involved in the case study, (2) there was enough time for interaction between the various sites, moderated in a way to support this, and (3) the presenters were familiar with the strategies for engaging the remote sites.

Conclusions from the PASGeP Initiative

The series is in its third year, and has maintained high levels of participation from all sites while drawing interest from other academic centers both nationally and internationally, as well as the media. Moreover, the telehealth rounds have received recognition by the Faculty of Medicine, University of Toronto through the Colin Woolf Award to Dr Morris Freedman in 2008 for excellence in course coordination. Additional participating countries from time to time also include South Africa, Switzerland (World Health Organization), the United States, and Argentina. The PASGeP initiative demonstrates how the language of health can be a bridge to communication and collaboration between countries that may not normally engage with each other, by focusing on common needs through continuing education. The adoption of health as a framework for building collaboration between countries as a bridge to peace is already being considered by some countries as a means of driving foreign policy, and PASGeP experience suggests that such a policy on the part of governments could be a fruitful investment.[32,33] Moreover, it is a testament to the process when Arabs and Israelis are heard describing each other not just as colleagues but as friends.

SUMMARY

Success in telemedicine is dependent on a wide variety of factors including strong institutional support, a solid business model,[34–38] enthusiastic and dedicated personnel, and continued acceptance and adoption of telemedicine worldwide. As with any other health care service, the keys to success will vary for each program, and the particular circumstances under which it is created and in which it operates. The lessons learned from those programs that have been able to succeed and become at least partially self-sustaining will, it is hoped, allow more telemedicine and telehealth programs to grow and provide more efficient and effective health care to patients throughout the world. In the clinical specialty of otolaryngology, these basic principles have led to the introduction of new technologies and new programs in recent years, and they are likely to continue to grow as models and options continue to expand.[39–42]

REFERENCES

1. Bashshur RL, Shannon GW. History of telemedicine. New York: Mary Ann Liebert, Inc.; 2009.
2. Norris AC. Essentials of telemedicine and telecare. West Sussex (England): John Wiley & Sons, Ltd; 2002.
3. Digital Imaging and Communications in Medicine (DICOM). Available at: http://medical.nema.org/. Accessed March 29, 2010.
4. Siegel E, Krupinski E, Samei E. Digital mammography image quality: image display. J Am Coll Radiol 2006;3(8):615–27.
5. Van Moore A, Allen B, Campbell SC. Report of the ACR task force on international teleradiology. J Am Coll Radiol 2005;2(2):121–5.
6. Guidelines for the surgical practice of telemedicine. SAGES (Society of American Gastrointestinal and Endoscopic Surgeons); 2004. Available at: http://www.sages.org/sagespublication.php?doc=21. Accessed March 29, 2010.
7. American Telemedicine Association. Core standards for telemedicine operations. Available at: http://www.americantelemed.org/files/public/standards/CoreStandards_withCOVER.pdf. Accessed March 29, 2010.
8. Krupinski E, Burdick A, Pak H. American Telemedicine Association's practice guidelines for teledermatology. Telemed J E Health 2007;14(3):289–302.
9. American Telemedicine Association. Telehealth practice recommendations for diabetic retinopathy. Telemed J E Health 2004;10(4):469–82.
10. American Telemedicine Association. Guidelines for telepathology. Available at: http://www.americantelemed.org/i4a/ams/amsstore/category.cfm?category_id=2. Accessed March 29, 2010.
11. American Telemedicine Association. Practice guidelines for videoconferencing-based telemental. Available at: http://www.americantelemed.org/files/public/standards/PracticeGuidelinesforVideoconferencing-Based%20TelementalHealth.pdf. Accessed March 29, 2010.
12. Kokesh J, Ferguson S, Patricoski C, et al. Traveling an audiologist to provide otolaryngology care using store-and-forward telemedicine. Telemed J E Health 2009;15(8):758–63.
13. Dorrian C, Ferguson J, Ah-See K, et al. Head and neck cancer assessment by flexible endoscopy and telemedicine. J Telemed Telecare 2009;15(3):118–21.
14. Xu CQ, Smith AC, Scuffman PA, et al. A cost minimization analysis of a telepaediatric otolaryngology service. BMC Health Serv Res 2008;8:30.
15. Weinstein RS, Lopez AM, Krupinski EA, et al. Integrating telemedicine and telehealth: putting it all together. In: Latifi R, editor. Current principles and practices of telemedicine and e-health. Washington, DC: IOS Press; 2008. p. 23–38.
16. Ackerman MJ, Filart R, Burgess LP, et al. Developing next-generation telehealth tools and technologies: patients, systems, and data perspectives. Telemed J E Health 2010;16(1):93–5.
17. Krupinski EA, Hughes AM, Barker GP, et al. Fluctuations in telemedicine case volume: correlation with personnel turnover rates. Telemed J E Health 2003; 9(4):369–73.
18. Puskin DS, Cohen Z, Ferguson AS, et al. Implementation and evaluation of telehealth tools and technologies. Telemed J E Health 2010;16(1):96–102.

19. Krupinski EA, Charness N, Demiris G, et al. Roundtable discussion: human factors in telemedicine. Telemed J E Health 2008;14(10):1024–30.
20. Burroughs CM, Wood FB. Measuring the difference: guide to planning and evaluating health information outreach. Bethesda (MD): National Library of Medicine; 2000.
21. Telehealth Adoption Toolkits. Available at: http://www.telehealthresourcecenter. org/toolbox.php. Accessed March 29, 2010.
22. Rowe N, Morley S, Krupinski EA. Ten-year experience of a private nonprofit telepsychiatry service. Telemed J E Health 2008;14(10):1078–86.
23. Krupinski EA. High-volume teleradiology service: focus on radiologist and patient satisfaction. In: Kumar S, Krupinski E, editors. Teleradiology. Berlin: Springer; 2008. p. 243–52.
24. Maffei R, Hudson Y, Dunn K. Telemedicine for urban uninsured: a pilot framework for specialty care planning for sustainability. Telemed J E Health 2008;14(9):925–31.
25. Barker GP, Krupinski EA, McNeely RA, et al. The Arizona Telemedicine Program business model. J Telemed Telecare 2005;11(8):397–402.
26. Khan S, Snyder HW, Rathke AM, et al. Is there a successful business case for telepharmacy? Telemed J E Health 2008;14(3):235–44.
27. Davalos ME, French MT, Burdick AE, et al. Economic evaluation of telemedicine: review of the literature and research guidelines for benefit-cost analysis. Telemed J E Health 2009;15(10):933–48.
28. Gagnon MP, Duplantie J, Fortin JP, et al. Implementing telehealth to support medical practice in rural/remote regions: what are the conditions for success? Implement Sci 2006;1(1):e18.
29. Skinner HA, Abdeen Z, Abdeen H, et al. Promoting Arab and Israeli cooperation: peacebuilding through health initiatives. Lancet 2005;365(9466):1274–7.
30. Noyek AM, Skinner H, Davis D, et al. Building bridges of understanding through continuing education and professional development of Arabs and Israelis. J Contin Educ Health Prof 2005;25(2):198–209.
31. Skinner HA, Sriharan A. Building cooperation through health initiatives: an Arab and Israeli case study. Confl Health 2007;1(1):e8.
32. Horton R. Health as an instrument of foreign policy. Lancet 2007;369(9564): 806–7.
33. Sambunjak D, Simunovic VJ. Peace through medical education in Bosnia and Herzegovina. Lancet 2007;369(9565):905.
34. Le Goff-Pronost M, Sicotte C. The added value of thorough economic evaluation of telemedicine networks. Eur J Health Econ 2010;11(1):45–55.
35. Wade VA, Karnon J, Elshaug AG, et al. A systematic review of economic analyses of telehealth services using real time video communications. BMC Health Serv Res 2010;10:233.
36. Demaerschalk BM, Hwang HM, Leung G. Cost analysis review of stroke centers, telestroke, and rt-PA. Am J Manag Care 2010;16(7):537–44.
37. Spaulding R, Belz N, DeLurgio S, et al. Cost savings of telemedicine utilization for child psychiatry in a rural Kansas community. Telemed J E Health 2010;16(8): 867–71.
38. Garrelts JC, Gagnon M, Eisenberg C, et al. Impact of telepharmacy in a multihospital health system. Am J Health Syst Pharm 2010;67(17):1456–62.
39. Choi H, Park IH, Yoon HG, et al. Wireless patient monitoring system for patients with nasal obstruction. Telemed J E Health 2011;17(1):46–9.
40. Boedeker BH, Bernhagen M, Miller DJ, et al. The combined use of Skype and the STORZ CMAC video laryngoscope in field intubation training with the Nebraska National Air Guard. Stud Health Technol Inform 2011;163:83–5.

41. Wormald RN, Moran RJ, Reilly RB, et al. Performance of an automated, remote system to detect vocal fold paralysis. Ann Otol Rhinol Laryngol 2008;117(11): 834–8.

42. Montgomery-Downs HE, Ramadan HH, Clawges HC, et al. Digital oral photography for pediatric tonsillar kypertrophy grading. Int J Pediatr Otorhinolaryngol 2011;75(6):841–3.

Consumer-Directed Telehealth

Cameron D. Norman, PhD

KEYWORDS

- Telehealth • Telemedicine • Patient-directed health care
- Consumer-directed health care • Health technology
- Mobile medicine • eHealth

Key Points

- Consumer-oriented telehealth bridges the gap between traditional medical informatics and public engagement in health care.
- The manner in which consumer-oriented telehealth is organized is along 3 orders that go from a simple, technology-based model (first order), to one in which technologies complement one another in providing information and services (second order), to one in which the technology is embedded as an essential part of a larger program (third order).
- To fully engage with this new form of telehealth, the public (patients) and health care professionals alike require new skills and knowledge that evolve along with the technology. This skills set, or eHealth literacy, represents an amalgam of generic and context-specific skills required to use technology effectively to address health issues in practice.
- Although technology is often highlighted as the focus of telehealth, it is human skill and the ability to work together that is the critical factor in determining the success of efforts to use information technology effectively to support health service delivery.
- Web 2.0 and social media now allow anyone with basic Internet skills to create, distribute, and modify content online, which is fundamentally changing the way communication is made through technology and the roles that both the public and health professionals play, introducing new opportunities for engagement and ethical challenges.

What if physical space and time were no longer limiting factors influencing access to health care? What if those who were ill or seeking the best health information or advice could do so in their local community instead of having to go somewhere else, sometimes never having to leave their own home? Telehealth services provide the means for anyone with access to simple technologies to receive care, learn about health

---

Peter A. Silverman Global eHealth Program, Dalla Lana School of Public Health, University of Toronto, 155 College Street, Room 586, Toronto, ON M5B2P7, Canada
E-mail address: cameron.norman@utoronto.ca

Otolaryngol Clin N Am 44 (2011) 1289–1296
doi:10.1016/j.otc.2011.08.005
0030-6665/11/$ – see front matter © 2011 Elsevier Inc. All rights reserved.

issues, and engage with other citizens (patients, providers and policy makers alike) at times and locations that are convenient and safe. This is not a utopian vision, but a reality for a growing number of people throughout the world, and something that has remarkable potential to support otolaryngology. Telehealth, the application of information and communication technologies to connect people to health resources, is a relatively new field of practice and research and has traditionally focused on connecting health care centers together; however, the rapid expansion of consumer-oriented tools and technologies beginning with the World Wide Web has redefined telehealth as something equally suited to consumers.

HISTORY AND DEFINITIONS OF TELEHEALTH

The information and communication technology boom that took place in the latter part of the twentieth century opened up new avenues for delivering information directly to consumers on demand through the telephone, computer screen, and mobile handset. This expansion of tools designed to facilitate communication provided opportunities to extend health care beyond the traditional settings like clinics and hospitals into places where people lived, worked, and played. It also offered an opportunity to capitalize on the growing interest in health education and health promotion,[1–3] providing means to support the public directly in self-care and prevention activities by linking primary care and specialized medicine with community/public health.

The Canadian Society for Telehealth (now part of COACH: Canada's Health Informatics Association) defines this field as follows:

> Telehealth has been defined as the use of information and communications technologies (ICTs), to deliver health services and transmit health information over both long and short distances. Telehealth helps eliminate distance barriers and improve equitable access to services that often would otherwise not be available in remote and rural communities. It is about transmitting voice, data, images, and information rather than moving patients or health practitioners and educators.
>
> Telehealth can best be described as the sharp end of e-health. It is where the information or data generated through the related discipline of health informatics is used in some form of direct (eg, one on one) or indirect (eg, Web site) interaction with a well citizen, ill patient, or fellow health care provider in any location.[4]

As the definition suggests, telehealth and eHealth are similar to each in other in many ways. eHealth has struggled with creating a definition, with multiple versions having been introduced in the leading journal in the field.[5–10] Consumer-directed telehealth adds a new element to this discussion, by focusing less on the informatics components emphasized in the discourse on eHealth applications, and more on the experience of the tools themselves and their impact on health knowledge, attitudes, behavior, and skills. The earliest study citing consumer-directed telehealth appeared in 2003,[11] with the first explicit use of the term appearing in 2006.[12] Since then, telehealth has continued to be explored as a means of addressing problems posed by distance, cost, and health care coverage.

Unlike most traditional telehealth services, which are focused on supporting or augmenting institutional-based health care activities, consumer-directed telehealth activities are less tied to settings and more to individuals. Peer-to-peer networking is a central feature of consumer-directed telehealth services, characterized by an individual practitioner, peer support resource, or third-party content provider to connect directly to the consumer without requiring any institutional or professional intermediary. Consumer-directed telehealth reaches people where they are physically, technologically, educationally, and in terms of psychosocial readiness.

CONSUMER-DIRECTED TELEHEALTH: 3 ORDERS

Consumer-directed telehealth may be viewed as comprising 3 orders[13]:

First order: stand-alone
Second order: complementary
Third order: integrated.

These 3 orders are discussed in this article, drawing on examples from the literature, particularly tobacco control, in which a large body of work on consumer-based telehealth exists[14] and where there is a high level of relevance to otolaryngologists.

First-order Consumer Telehealth

A first-order telehealth service is designed to operate independently of any other resource or application. A first-order resource may include Web sites, message services (eg, short message service [SMS]), or peer-to-peer interaction opportunities designed solely to function on its own, without any additional services required to add value. These resources may refer to other services via links to Web sites or reference sources like books or telephone services; however, these additional elements are not considered essential for the telehealth service to function. This factor is what distinguishes first-order telehealth resources from second-order or third-order ones, which are discussed in greater detail later.

First-order resources represents the simplest application of consumer-directed telehealth and can comprise free or low-cost tools to more sophisticated paid models; however, the consistent factor is that the service is based solely on a technological platform. Within the range of different technological options, this platform could be a Web site, a text or video message, an audio or video podcast, streaming media, or voice-enabled delivery system. Although these services may facilitate some form of live interaction, the scale and scope of services may be limited during certain hours. In the case of social media such as social networking platforms, in which the value is almost exclusively drawn from the users of the site, the opportunities are immense and diverse.

Examples of a first-order telehealth resource for consumers include Web sites that provide smoking cessation services[14,15] or providing a text-message service to do the same.[16,17] In both cases, the telehealth services are self-contained and require no additional resources to be effective.

Second-order Consumer Telehealth

A second-order consumer telehealth service is one that is deployed in conjunction with another type of resource (eg, telephone helpline) or face-to-face clinical intervention. Second-order consumer telehealth services are different from first-order ones in that they are designed to play a complementary role to other forms of service. This role could mean a Web site or Web appendix to complement a printed book or a public health information hotline that is used alongside of other campaigns delivered in the community.

A second-order consumer telehealth service can also be designed as a cluster of different telehealth resources that offer different ways to connect to the same information. One example of this is the Canadian Cancer Society (CCS) Smokers' Helpline Web site (http://www.smokershelpline.ca), which follows the previous smoking cessation examples. The Smokers' Helpline was originally developed as a telephone-based telehealth resource; however, with the growth of the World Wide Web, the CCS opted to expand the service to the Internet and later to text messaging and use of social network tools like Facebook. The CCS Smokers' Helpline is staffed by trained smoking cessation professionals who provide information, quitting tips, and links to self-help resources and health services that can aid individuals looking to stop using tobacco or who wish to support someone else.

The use of different modalities of service offers the CCS a means of reaching people through methods that fit their lifestyle that acknowledges genuine resource constraints. For example, the telephone support service is available mostly during the day, with limited availability in the evenings. Although the Web site is available 24 hours a day, it favors those with access to computers, which is where the text-messaging service is most effective because it can reach people who are not able to go online. Whenever possible, the various modes provide overlapping services that complement one another to provide the greatest amount of reach and opportunity for the public (or patients) to engage with the telehealth resource.

Third-order Consumer Telehealth

A third-order consumer-directed telehealth service is one that is fully integrated into an existing program of activity. Unlike second-order interventions, third-order consumer telehealth services are embedded within a larger programming structure in which the resource is not viewed as complementary or stand-alone, but integral to the activities performed using different methods. Third-order telehealth services require a more sophisticated approach to service delivery and enhanced coordination above that of most activities in a first-order and second-order intervention or resource. Because they are embedded within other programs, a level of coherence and synergy between the different components is necessary for the service to operate effectively. However, the result of these efforts can produce a program that is more detailed, intense, and able to be tailored to the needs of specific consumers or conditions. Computer-based clinical assessments can serve as a starting point for such third-order interventions,[18] by providing a means of linking patient data about a visit before the clinical encounter.

One organization that has developed an array of tools and resources using third-order telehealth is TakingITGlobal, a Toronto-based nongovernmental organization that seeks to engage young adults and educators using new technologies. TakingIT-Global's integrated virtual classroom initiative for providing health education and promotion support to teachers (TiGEd) provides an example of a third-order consumer-directed telehealth intervention directed to secondary schoolteachers in countries around the globe.[19] TiGEd features a series of virtual classrooms on a variety of health topics including food security, human immunodeficiency virus/AIDS stigma, and tobacco control. For example, *The Virtual Classroom on Tobacco Control* was cocreated in partnership with the Youth Voices Research Group at the University of Toronto. *The Virtual Classroom* is designed for both young smokers and nonsmokers (ages 12–24 years) and intended for delivery in educational settings.[20] This school-based telehealth resource is designed to provide interactive resources to support the teaching of health in secondary schools, either through electronic connectivity with students directly accessing the Web site, or by providing teachers with a means to download materials for use in face-to-face lectures. This strategy enables the resource to be used in areas of high connectivity and low.

The Virtual Classroom was built around a comprehensive telehealth resource, *The Smoking Zine*,[21] which was evaluated in a large, school-based randomized controlled trial.[22] *The Smoking Zine*, originally designed as a first-order consumer-directed telehealth resource, has been since modified into second-order and third-order interventions to suit a variety of circumstances and settings. Taken together, *The Virtual Classroom* provides a means of offering multiple options for teachers and takes advantage of the strengths of different modes of communicating health information to consumers.

Facilitators and Limitations

Literacy

One of the most overlooked issues in telehealth is literacy, particularly when the delivery mechanism includes text.[23] Literacy in the case of telehealth is a complex process that goes beyond simple reading and writing and includes the basic skills needed to operate the tools and software, and the ability to place health information into the proper context, a skill set called eHealth literacy.[24] eHealth literacy is a composite skill that is made up of 6 literacies organized into 2 central types: analytical (traditional, media, information) and context-specific (computer, scientific, health). These basic skills are described in the following paragraphs.

The analytical component involves skills that are applicable to a broad range of information sources irrespective of the topic or context, whereas the context-specific component relies on more situation-specific skills. For example, analytical skills can be applied as much to shopping or researching a term paper as they can to health.

Context-specific skills are just as important; however, their application is more likely to be contextualized within a specific problem domain or circumstance. Thus, computer literacy is dependent on what type of technology is being used and its operating system, as well as its intended application.

Scientific literacy is applied to problems in which research-related information is presented, just as health literacy is contextualized to health issues as opposed to shopping for a new television set. Yet, both analytical and context-specific skills are required to fully engage with electronic health resources.

This complex set of overlapping skills is one of the central challenges facing consumer-directed telehealth. Drawing on the author's experience evaluating telehealth programs in continuing education and health promotion, the most salient challenge in connecting any remote site to another is ensuring that local expertise is available to manage the connection and tools on each side of the transmission.[25]

Technical Issues

As with any system that relies on technology, consumer telehealth is beset with both technical and human limitations. Bandwidth constraints and wireless coverage are some of the major barriers to using these tools. Technical connectivity is another. Without reliable high-speed broadband access, only the most basic telehealth services are likely to be successful. The one exception to this is in the area of text-messaging (SMS) enabled telehealth services,[26,27] in which information can be delivered reliably, inexpensively, and efficiently using technologies that are widespread and often reach into areas where broadband access is nonexistent.

Compatibility is another issue that limits telehealth. Although it may be easy to select technologies that meet the standards of the day, developing strategies to enable these tools to evolve over time in a manner that maintains their compatibility is a different problem. One of these issues is selecting between tools and devices that are platform-dependent or vendor-dependent. For example, Apple's operating systems (OSs) are not designed for use on any computer other than a Mac, whereas the

Blackberry OS is designed only for devices manufactured by Research in Motion. Vendor-specific options provide stability and limit flexibility.

An alternative option is to move toward open-access and open-source software platforms. Open source refers to the ability for others to access the source-programming code that underlies the telehealth resource, which includes the potential to have this code copied, modified, or replaced. These solutions, such as the Firefox Web browser, Linux OS, or Google's Android mobile platform, are often more responsive and innovative than their closed-source peers; however, such open-source models are also vulnerable to bugs and instabilities in early releases.

One example of how this model has worked in telehealth and eHealth is the *Journal of Medical Internet Research* (http://www.jmir.org), which has become the highest-impact publication in eHealth and the second highest within health services research within 10 years of its launch. Although this is impressive for an author-funded publication, *JMIR* has gone so far as to offer its entire journal publishing platform for free to anyone wishing to adopt it to create a new journal using the source code created by the developer.

Web 2.0

The concept of Web 2.0 was coined by Internet business leader Tim O'Reilly to describe the move from a largely static form of the Internet in which content developers had to possess some technical programming language to build a Web site. Although the basic Web-programming skills were easy to acquire, they did pose a barrier to those not interested in programming. The advent of Web 2.0 changed that situation. It enabled people to generate content online with limited knowledge of the mechanisms behind the programming. Thus, if you could use a word processor or Web browser, you could add content. Web 2.0 tools include social networking Web sites (eg, Facebook), wikis (editable Web forms for collaborative writing), and direct-to-Internet publishing such as blogs or microblog services (eg, Twitter).

Included in this Web 2.0 revolution is the concept of social media. Social media is the term used to describe content the value of which is derived from social interaction in an electronic space. Social networks such as Facebook and MySpace or micro-blogging networks like Twitter are examples of social media. This technology represents a radical departure for those using telehealth services, given the emphasis on interactive content. Social media and Web 2.0 represent a fundamental shift in how and where power and influence are exerted in the relationships in health. In educational environments using Web 2.0, no longer is content generated and passively absorbed by students, it is cocreated and recreated as learner-generated content, and feedback adds to the initial presentation. This type of interaction requires that teachers acknowledge the skills and limitations of their audience as they jointly become prosumers (producers and consumers of content).[28] The fundamental change in using these second-generation Web tools is not so much the technology, but adopting a position of openness and flexibility in using it and engaging with users regardless of their social position. Social media is about relationships, connectivity, and knowledge and less about social position and hierarchy, which often serve as a foundation for much of traditional medical environments.

Mobile Connectivity

Mobile applications for telehealth represent the future of the field, with mobile devices representing the greatest area of growth in the consumer market worldwide.[29] Most new mobile handset telephone devices are Web-enabled, providing a rich-text means of communicating when appropriate wireless networks exist. Mobile tools provide new ways of getting information to consumers in settings that are often difficult to wire for Internet or where reliable connectivity is lacking. Mobile devices are also typically more affordable that desktop or laptop computers, providing an economical as well as portable means of creating or consuming content.

The introduction of the iPad and other tablet and mobile reading devices such as the Amazon Kindle, Blackberry Playbook, and Sony e-reader has opened up a new possibility for consumer-directed telehealth. These tools require relatively little knowledge of computers and cost less than typical laptops or desktops, yet have more functionality than mobile phones and are easier to read from or view rich-content materials like videos and photographs/images. As these technologies develop and their cost decreases, the opportunities to create truly sharable computing for delivering consumer-directed telehealth interventions will increase.

SUMMARY

Consumer-directed telehealth is an emerging area of practice, research, and general innovation that has tremendous benefits for otolaryngology. As mobile computing introduces more high-resolution devices to support clinical practice and communication, the opportunities for consumer-directed telehealth will increase on many levels. Current trends suggest that mobile computing and greater use of video and pictures to support peer-to-peer communication (and telehealth opportunities) will become more widespread than ever before. As tablet computers such as the iPad proliferate and costs decrease, it is reasonable to expect that the reliance on paper records and materials to support learning and patient care will decrease as well, moving health care providers and institutions to more interactive, digital, high-definition options that are stored electronically.

As these opportunities increase, so too will the demands on otolaryngologists and their support teams to continue learning about electronic tools to better engage their patients and their peers. eHealth literacy is likely to be a core competence for everyone involved in consumer-related education, interventions, and service. With this literacy will come the ability to make strategic decisions about what the most appropriate order of service is needed for each case and how best to leverage the tremendous opportunities provided by new technologies to enhance the health experience for everyone, regardless of where they are.

REFERENCES

1. International Conference on Primary Health Care. Declaration of Alma-Ata. Alma-Ata (USSR): International Conference on Primary Health Care; 1978.
2. Ottawa charter of health promotion. Geneva (CH): World Health Organization; 1996. p. 4.
3. The Bangkok charter for health promotion in a globalized world. Bangkok (Thailand): World Health Organization; 2005. p. 1–6.
4. Canadian Society of Telehealth. About telehealth. Ottawa (ON): COACH: Canada's Health Informatics Association; 2010.
5. Ahern KD, Kreslake MJ, Phalen MJ. What is eHealth (6): perspectives on the evolution of eHealth research. J Med Internet Res 2006;8:e4.
6. Della Mea V. What is eHealth (2): the death of telemedicine? J Med Internet Res 2001;22:e22.
7. Eysenbach G. What is eHealth? J Med Internet Res 2001;1:e20.

8. Jones R, Rogers R, Roberts J, et al. What is eHealth (5): a research agenda for eHealth through stakeholder consultation and policy context review. J Med Internet Res 2005;7:e54.

9. Oh H, Rizo C, Enkin M, et al. What is eHealth (3): a systematic review of published definitions. J Med Internet Res 2005;7:11.

10. Pagliari C, Sloan D, Gregor P, et al. What is eHealth (4): a scoping exercise to map the field. J Med Internet Res 2005;7:e9.

11. Bynum AB, Cranford CO, Irwin CA, et al. Participant satisfaction in an adult tele-health education program using interactive compressed video delivery methods in rural Arkansas. J Rural Health 2003;19:218–22.

12. Doswell JT. Consumer telehealth for improving care for the uninsured: a human rights need. Boston: American Public Health Association; 2006.

13. Norman CD. Using information technology to support smoking-related behaviour change: web-assisted tobacco interventions. Smoking Cessation Rounds 2007; 1:1–6.

14. Norman CD, Mcintosh S, Selby P, et al. Web-assisted tobacco interventions: empowering change in the global fight for the public's (e)health. J Med Internet Res 2008;10:e48.

15. Etter JF. A list of the most popular smoking cessation web sites and a comparison of their quality. Nicotine Tob Res 2006;8:S27–34.

16. Rodgers A, Corbett T, Bramley D, et al. Do u smoke after txt? Results of a randomized trial of smoking cessation using mobile phone text messaging. Tobacco Control 2005;10:1–7.

17. Whittaker R, Maddison R, Mcrobbie H, et al. A multimedia mobile phone-based youth smoking cessation intervention: findings from content development and piloting studies. J Med Internet Res 2008;10:e49.

18. Ahmad F, Hogg-Johnson S, Stewart DE, et al. Computer-assisted screening for intimate partner violence and control: a randomized trial. Ann Intern Med 2009; 151:93–102.

19. TakingITGlobal. Toronto (ON): TiGEd Homepage; 2010.

20. TakingITGlobal. Toronto (ON): Virtual Classroom on Tobacco Control; 2010.

21. Youth voices research group. Toronto (ON): The Smoking Zine; 2010.

22. Norman CD, Maley O, Li X, et al. Using the Internet to assist smoking prevention and cessation in schools: a randomized, controlled trial. Health Psychol 2008;27: 799–810.

23. Schmeida M, McNeal R. The telehealth divide: disparities in searching public health information online. J Health Care Poor Underserved 2007;18:637–47.

24. Norman CD, Skinner HA. eHealth literacy: essential skills for consumer health in a networked world. J Med Internet Res 2006;8:e9.

25. Norman CD, Sriharan A, Freedman M, et al. Delivery and evaluation of a video-conference-based program for diagnosis and treatment education linking Canada and the Middle East. Vancouver (BC) Canada: CME Congress; 2008.

26. Bjerke TN, Kummervold PE, Christiansen EK, et al. "It made me feel connected"—an exploratory study on the use of mobile SMS in follow-up care for substance abusers. J Addict Nurs 2008;19:195–200.

27. Cocosila M, Archer N, Yuan Y. Adoption of SMS for health adherence: a consumer perspective. Conference Paper/Presentation. 2009 World Congress on privacy, security, trust and the management of e-Business. Saint John (NB) Canada; 2009.

28. Wurman RS. Information anxiety 2. Indianapolis (IN): QUE; 2001.

29. The mobile internet report. New York: Morgan Stanley; 2009.

Teleaudiology

Mark Krumm, PhD[a,b], Mark J. Syms, MD[c,d],*

KEYWORDS

• Teleaudiology • Telehealth • Remote computing
• Early hearing detection

While telehealth technology has been used for over a century, teleaudiology research began in the mid-1990s. Teleaudiology research in this era incorporated video oto-scopy,[1,2] hearing aid fittings using remote computing technology,[3] and synchronous applications with hearing testing.[4] Over the past 10 years, teleaudiology research has been limited until recently, when several publications describing different systems dedicated to hearing assessment and rehabilitation were published. The catalyst behind the growth of teleaudiology was due to the advent of low-cost (but effective) Web cameras and affordable broad-band connectivity. At the same time, audiology equipment for diagnosis, hearing aid fittings, and for cochlear implants became increasingly computerized. Consequently, clinicians were able to interface computer-ized audiology equipment with telehealth technology to provide a variety of hearing health care services to underserved communities. Teleaudiology is still in its early stages, and considerable research is necessary before widespread audiology services can be confidently offered using telehealth technology.

Asynchronous data transfer is most commonly used today by hearing health care professionals. Specifically, asynchronous technology is used when information such as tympanograms, audiograms, auditory brainstem response recordings, or video-otoscopy images are transmitted via E-mail or by fax. Asynchronous studies have been published evaluating the efficacy of telehealth with tympanometry, video-nystagmography (VNG), and video-otoscopy.[1,5,6] In addition, E-mail communication has been used to deliver cognitive–behavioral therapy for tinnitus treatment[7] and for counseling new hearing aid users.[8]

One appealing asynchronous application is self-assessment of hearing sensitivity. Presently, self-assessment procedures involving hearing testing online appear to

Financial Disclosure: Mark Krumm: Nothing to disclose. Mark J. Syms is a shareholder of Cochlear Corporation and Sonova Holdings.
[a] North East Ohio AuD Consortium (NOAC), Kent State University, A104 Music and Speech Building, Kent, OH 44242, USA
[b] Department of Speech Pathology and Audiology, Kent State University, A104 Music and Speech Building, Kent, OH 44242, USA
[c] Neurotology, Barrow Neurological Institute, 2910 North 3rd Avenue, Phoenix, AZ 85013, USA
[d] Arizona Ear Center, 2627 North 3rd Street Suite 201, Phoenix, AZ 85004, USA
* Corresponding author. Arizona Ear Center, 2627 North 3rd Street Suite 201, Phoenix, AZ 85004.
E-mail address: m.syms@arizonaear.com

Otolaryngol Clin N Am 44 (2011) 1297–1304
doi:10.1016/j.otc.2011.08.006
0030-6665/11/$ – see front matter © 2011 Elsevier Inc. All rights reserved.

suffer from questionable calibration, poor validation, and the lack of control over environmental noise levels. However, phone-based hearing screening programs using speech in noise stimuli as described by Smits and colleagues[9] have been validated and overcome many of the calibration issues associated with pure tone testing over the phone.

Synchronous services are characterized by the clinician delivering services to clients in real time or live. Interactive video is typically used with synchronous services to observe patient responses to stimuli and to assure clinicians that audiometric equipment (transducer, probes, and electrodes) are properly placed. Interactive video may be provided by a laptop Web camera or by a dedicated camera system that is interfaced directly to the computer network. While interactive video can require substantial bandwidth, the benefits are obvious, providing the clinician and patient with services that are essentially face to face.

Audiologists may use 2 models of synchronous telehealth models. The first model is the traditional telehealth model in which only interactive video is used to implement services. This model requires the extensive use of high-quality interactive video for the clinician to supervise technician test procedures at the remote site. Once the technician obtains patient data, the clinician will typically provide a diagnosis and recommend management.

Synchronous teleaudiology has already been used successfully by Marincovich in the mid-1990s to provide hearing evaluations and hearing aid fittings in a rural region of California (Peter Marincovich, PhD, April 2009). In implementing this model, the technician must be trained well enough to administer, but not necessarily interpret, audiology test results. Rather, interpretation and counseling are done by the hearing health care professional using interactive video with the patient. This is an effective solution when the technician turnover is low, and ongoing technician training is possible. Also, the traditional model has the benefit of comparatively modest technology requirements.

Another form of synchronous audiology services incorporates remote control, in so that clinicians can test patients at distant sites. This is a reasonable telehealth strategy to consider, as many audiology systems are computerized and use a Windows operating system. Therefore, a clinician at 1 site can control computerized audiology equipment at a distant site using application sharing (or remote computing) software through a network, modem, or the Internet. In essence, remote computing creates a method that extends the hands of the clinician from 1 clinic site to another (**Fig. 1**). The greatest advantage to this method is that a technician is not required to do testing at the patient site. Therefore, technician skills and training are not critical. However, a technician is still required to do tasks such as providing patient basic instructions, transducer placement, and otoscopy. Additionally, he or she must have some skills in running the computer at the patient site. **Figs. 2** and **3** provide an example of equipment that can be used at the evaluator and patient locations.

Using this paradigm, investigators have employed synchronous protocols to administer a variety of common hearing tests to subjects including pure tone, speech, otoacoustic emissions, and the auditory brainstem-evoked response.[10–16] In addition, synchronous technology has been used to program hearing aids and cochlear implants.[17–23] The model for delivery is illustrated in **Fig. 4**. Remote computing technology presently requires further validation but has been used successfully to administer hearing tests over considerable distances.[10–13] The fiscal limitation of these applications is due to the need for personnel participating in the care at both locations. Currently, reimbursement for audiologic services is difficult with 1 provider involved in the care. The addition of personnel at the remote site makes the financial viability

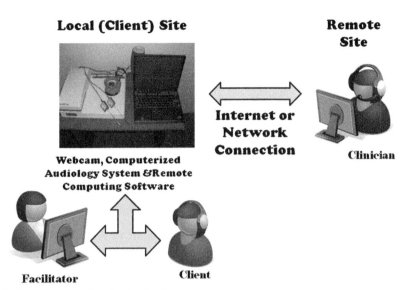

Fig. 1. A synchronous hearing test system.

less favorable. Further clinical and financial validation is needed to increase the adoption of teleaudiology.

HYBRID MODEL

While the sole use of asynchronous or synchronous technology appears to be reasonable in some circumstances, clinicians should consider the most efficient system to deliver telehealth services. In many cases, a combination of synchronous and asynchronous technology will yield the best solution for hearing health care services. This

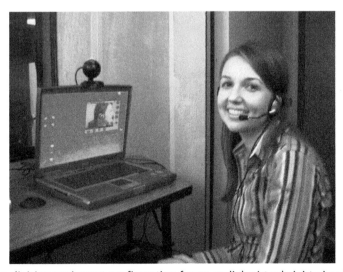

Fig. 2. The clinician equipment configuration for an audiologist administering telehealth services. Note only a computer (with remote computing software) and a video system (either web cam or dedicated video) are required at the clinician site.

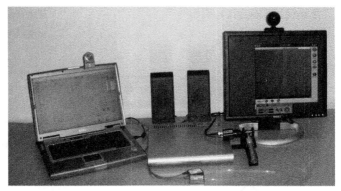

Fig. 3. Equipment required at the patient site. For remote computing purposes, a computer, Web camera or dedicated camera, computerized audiometric equipment (an audiometer is pictured), video-otoscopy, immittance (not shown), and a LAN connection would permit basic teleaudiology services.

combination of technology is considered a hybrid model and is regularly used in successful telehealth programs. A recent study was published describing hybrid hearing screening services for young school-aged children.[6] The investigators of this study used interactive video via a Web camera to see the responses of children receiving hearing screenings. In addition, the investigators used remote computing to present pure tone stimuli at the school, an audiometer that was purposefully developed for telehealth applications and video-otoscopy interfaced to the Web camera. Tympanometry results were viewed via Web camera at the time of the screening, scanned into a computer at the end of the day, and then later sent via email to the investigators for final interpretation. One of the issues with research in teleaudiology is few authors are describing a complete battery of diagnostic hearing services. In all likelihood, hybrid systems will be used in the future to offer complete hearing services.

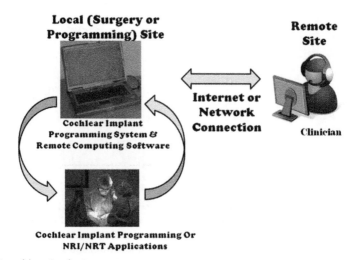

Fig. 4. A cochlear implant care.

EMERGING TELEAUDIOLOGY
Telehealth and Infant Applications

In all likelihood, telehealth will be increasingly used by practitioners involved with early hearing detection and intervention (EDHI) programs. In recent funding programs, the US government has encouraged statewide EDHI programs to use teleaudiology applications. This is not surprising, as EDHI program goals can be difficult to achieve due to inadequate professional expertise, lack of program planning, and insufficient funding.[24] Further, an EDHI program should exhibit continuity of services, up-to-date information, operate as a community-based health program, and provide accurate tracking information for newborns requiring further screening or assessment.[24] O'Neil and colleagues,[25] addressing similar EDHI issues, suggested new paradigms should be developed to ensure that each infant is provided needed services regardless of circumstances. Such a paradigm may incorporate telehealth services. However, telehealth has not been widely used to provide hearing screening or assessment services to infants.

Remote Computing Infant Hearing Assessment

Screening and diagnostic services are ordinarily administered using otoacoustic emissions (OAEs) or the auditory brainstem response (ABR). One intriguing aspect of ABR and OAEs systems is they are usually computer peripherals operated through desktop personal computers (PCs). Consequently, many ABR and OAE systems can be employed for both synchronous and asynchronous telehealth applications.

Synchronous computing applications for infant hearing screening seem to have at least 3 advantages. Specifically, when hearing screenings procedures cannot be accomplished face to face, a hearing heath care professional could conduct hearing screening from another location. Also, once personnel are trained to conduct infant hearing assessment in underserved area, these individuals can be mentored and supervised by a hearing health care professional in real time while screening clients. Another advantage to remote computing is that it can be used to observe practices at distant centers for quality control purposes. Such an application might be considered to achieve appropriate referral rates and to reduce excessive false positives.

Only 2 papers have been published concerning telehealth and OAEs and ABR in pediatric populations. One publication discussed theoretical pediatric applications of telehealth and otoacoustic emissions written by Krumm and colleagues.[26] This paper provided rationale, models, and pilot data supporting the use of telehealth technology with infant hearing screening programs.

In 2008, Krumm and colleagues described a study in which they used remote computing technology to record distortion product otoacoustic emissions (DPOAEs) and automated auditory brainstem audiometry response (AABR) data with infants.[13] Specifically, 30 infants ranging in age from 11 to 45 days (with an average age of 16 days) were seen for this study. Subjects recruited for this study did not pass prior DPOAE screening at birth and were being seen for rescreening at their regional medical hospital. Results obtained via face to face and via telehealth were essentially equal according to the authors. While most of the infants in this study were normal, the results suggest that synchronous (or a hybrid system) would provide reasonable support for EHDI programs lacking personnel expertise in underserved areas. **Fig. 5** is a screen capture of a synchronous session in which the child was receiving hearing evaluation with a DPOAE system.

It should be recognized that technicians are needed at the local (client) site to apply EOAE probes, ear phones, and electrodes to infants when actual hearing testing is

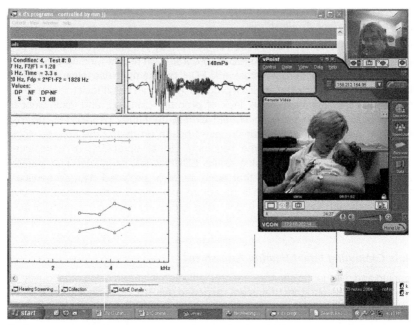

Fig. 5. Screen capture of a remote computing session in which DPOAEs are being measured in a young child.

conducted by telehealth. Also, technicians must be trained to adjust malfunctioning or improperly fitting screening probes, electrodes, or earphones during hearing screenings. So, further investigation examining the use of a trained assistant is necessary in future teleaudiology studies.

Much of the emphasis of recent publications has been dedicated discussing pure tone audiometry systems newly developed for telehealth purposes. The results of these and other publications generally describe only a single audiology service. While the outcomes of these studies are quite encouraging, telehealth researchers need to consider developing protocols employing a routine battery of diagnostic services. Also, most of the teleaudiology research has been administered to individuals with normal hearing. Clearly, validation must occur with significant numbers of individuals with hearing loss for teleaudiology to be useful. Finally, much of the research has been conducted under tightly controlled conditions rather than in the field with real consumers. Field-based research is needed to determine how well consumers are served with long-term teleaudiology services.

In addition to synchronous applications, employing asynchronous and hybrid telehealth models should also be for services and intervention services in underserved communities. Remote computing might prove valuable as a means to provide ongoing instruction to hearing screening assistants established in rural areas, particularly with EDHI services. Specifically, clinicians can mentor and monitor assistants using remote computing applications while viewing newborn hearing screenings in real time. These services would be dispensed with the goal of enhancing personnel expertise for newborn hearing screenings.

For clinicians contemplating telehealth applications, a few issues need to be reviewed. First of all, additional licensure or other certification may be needed to provide services in different regions and countries. It must also be recognized that few teleaudiology systems have been approved by the US Food and Drug Administration. This is a problematic issue that may ultimately limit telehealth services.

Reimbursement for telehealth services may be unclear, so funding sources must be identified before telehealth services are initiated. Also, while it is likely that most computerized audiology systems will work well for remote computing applications, clinicians must prototype prospective computerized audiology systems for the remote computing and asynchronous applications, to be assured that the telehealth technology will work as desired. Questionnaires should be provided to consumers who are served through telehealth services. With such planning, it is likely clinicians can extend their reach to patients hundreds or thousands of miles away.

REFERENCES

1. Birkmire-Peters DP, Peters LJ, Whitaker LA. A usability evaluation for telemedicine medical equipment: a case study. Telemed J 1999;5(2):209–12.
2. Sullivan R. Video otoscopy in audiologic practice. J Am Acad Audiol 1997;8: 447–67.
3. Fabry DA. Remote hearing aid fitting applications. Presented at the 8th Annual Mayo Clinic Audiology Videoconference. Mayo Center in Rochester, November, 1996.
4. Krumm M, Marincovich P, Hogarth B, et al. Providing audiological services through a telemedicine medium. Paper presented at the meeting of the American Academy of Audiology. San Diego, California, April, 2001.
5. Yates JT, Campbell KH. Audiovestibular education and services via telemedicine technologies. Semin Hear 2005;26:35–42.
6. Lancaster P, Krumm M, Ribera J. Remote hearing screenings via telehealth in a rural elementary school. Am J Audiol 2008;17(2):114–22.
7. Kaldo-Sandström V, Larsen HC, Andersson G. Internet-based cognitive–behavioral self-help treatment of tinnitus: clinical effectiveness and predictors of outcome. Am J Audiol 2004;13(2):185–92.
8. Laplante-Lévesque A, Pichora-Fuller MK, Gagné JP. Providing an internet-based audiological counseling programme to new hearing aid users: a qualitative study. Int J Audiol 2003;45:697–706.
9. Smits C, Kapteyn T, Houtgast T. Development and validation of an automatic speech-in-noise screening test by telephone. Int J Audiol 2004;43(1):15–28.
10. Krumm M, Ribera J, Klich R. Providing basic hearing tests using remote computing technology. J Telemed Telecare 2007;13(8):406–10.
11. Ribera J. Interjudge reliability and validation of telehealth applications of the hearing in noise test. Semin Hear 2005;26:13–8.
12. Swanepoel DW, Koekemoer D, Clark J. Intercontinental hearing assessment— a study in teleaudiology. J Telemed Telecare 2010;16(5):248–52.
13. Krumm M, Huffman T, Dick K, et al. Providing infant hearing screening using OAEs and ABR using telehealth technology. J Telemed Telecare 2008;14(2):102–4.
14. Choi J, Lee H, Park C, et al. PC-based teleaudiometry. Telemed J E Health 2007; 13(5):501–8.
15. Givens G, Elangovan S. Internet application to teleaudiology—"nothin' but net". Am J Audiol 2003;12:50–65.
16. Towers AD, Pisa J, Froelich TM, et al. The reliability of click-evoked and frequency-specific auditory brainstem response testing using telehealth technology. Semin Hear 2005;26:19–25.

17. Ferrari DV, Bernardez-Braga GR. Remote probe microphone measurement to verify hearing aid performance. J Telemed Telecare 2009;15:122–4.
18. Wesendahl T. Hearing aid fitting: application of telemedicine in audiology. Int Tinnitus J 2003;9(1):56–8.
19. Franck K, Pengelly M, Zerfoss S. Telemedicine offers remote cochlear implant programming. Volta Voices 2006;13(1):16–9.
20. Ramos A, Rodriguez C, Martinez-Beneyto P, et al. Use of telemedicine in the remote programming of cochlear implants. Acta Otolaryngol 2009;129:533–40.
21. Shapiro W, Huang T, Shaw T, et al. Remote intraoperative monitoring during cochlear implant surgery is feasible and efficient. Otol Neurotol 2008;29:495–8.
22. McElveen JT Jr, Blackburn EL, Green JD Jr, et al. Remote programming of cochlear implants: a telecommunications model. Otol Neurotol 2010;31(7): 1035–40.
23. Wesarg T, Wasowski A, Skarzynski H, et al. Remote fitting in Nucleus cochlear implant recipients. Acta Otolaryngol 2010;130(12):1379–88.
24. Mencher G, Davis A, Devoe S, et al. Universal neonatal screening: past, present, and future. Am J Audiol 2001;10:3–12.
25. O'Neal J, Finitzo T, Littman T. Neonatal hearing screening: followup and diagnosis. In: Roeser RJ, Valente M, Hosford-Dunn H, editors. Audiology diagnosis. New York: Thieme Medical Publishers; 2000. p. 527–44.
26. Krumm M, Ribera J, Schmiedge J. Using a telehealth medium for objective hearing testing: implications for supporting rural universal newborn hearing screening programs (UNHS). Semin Hear 2005;26(1):3–12.

Remote Management of Voice and Swallowing Disorders

Pauline A. Mashima, PhD[a,b],*, Janet E. Brown, MA[c]

KEYWORDS

• Telehealth • Telepractice • Telerehabilitation
• Speech-language pathology • Voice disorders • Dysphonia
• Swallowing disorders • Dysphagia

Speech-language pathologists (SLPs) are certified and licensed professionals who provide clinical services to optimize individuals' ability to communicate and swallow with the objective of improving their function and quality of life. SLPs collaborate with otolaryngologists to evaluate and treat individuals with communication and swallowing disorders associated with conditions such as neurologic diseases, head and neck cancer, benign laryngeal lesions, craniofacial anomalies, and hearing loss.

Access to speech-language pathology services is a significant problem in many geographic areas, due to a shortage of SLPs. According to the US Bureau of Labor Statistics, the demand for SLPs is expected to grow by 19% from 2008 to 2018.[1] A health care survey conducted by the American Speech-Language-Hearing Association (ASHA) in 2009 indicated that 25% of respondents had unfilled positions in their facility. The highest percentage of vacancies (36%) was in home health.[2] Although the rate of reported vacancies of SLPs in health care has decreased from its high of 40% in 2005,[3] these shortages are most likely to be felt in rural and underserved areas, which are also less likely to have SLPs specializing in voice and swallowing assessments and treatments.

The views expressed in this article are those of the authors and do not reflect the official policy or position of the Department of the Army, Department of Defense, or the US Government.
[a] Otolaryngology Service, Speech Pathology Section, Tripler Army Medical Center, 1 Jarrett White Road, Tripler AMC, Honolulu, HI 96859, USA
[b] Department of Communication Sciences and Disorders, University of Hawaii at Manoa, 1410 Lower Campus Road, Honolulu, HI 96822, USA
[c] Health Care Services in Speech-Language Pathology, American Speech-Language-Hearing Association, 2200 Research Boulevard, Rockville, MD 20850, USA
* Corresponding author. Otolaryngology Service, Speech Pathology Section, Tripler Army Medical Center, 1 Jarrett White Road, Tripler AMC, Honolulu, HI 96859.
E-mail address: pauline.mashima@amedd.army.mil

Key Points: REMOTE MANAGEMENT OF VOICE AND SWALLOWING DISORDERS

- Shortages of speech-language pathologists (SLPs), particularly in rural and remote areas, make telehealth a desirable means of accessing SLPs with specialties in voice and swallowing.

- Peripheral devices that can be used to support speech and swallowing services provided via telehealth include digital audio and video recording, otoscopes, endoscopes, fluoroscopes, and document cameras.

- Remote assessment facilitates decision making about the need for a follow-up visit, advancing the vocal rehabilitation program, and readiness for discharge.

- Voice treatment programs delivered via telehealth have been demonstrated to be comparable with in-person services where the audio and visual signals are adequate for the clinical application.

- Remote videofluoroscopic swallowing assessments show good agreement with on-site assessments and treatment recommendations where the visual image is adequate.

- Major barriers for the expanded use of telehealth by SLPs are licensure requirements for interstate practice and ineligibility to bill for telehealth services under Medicare Part B. Recognition and reimbursement by state Medicaid programs and private insurance are progressing slowly.

- Additional research is needed to investigate clinical and operational aspects of remote management of voice and swallowing disorders. Outcome measures including clinical effectiveness and clinician and patient satisfaction have been positive in the limited studies available.

The potential benefit of telehealth in speech-language pathology is significant in light of personnel shortages, decreasing technological costs, more widespread connectivity, an increasing demand for home health care, and changes in our nation's demographics with an expanding geriatric population more susceptible to communication and swallowing problems. In addition to improving accessibility to and increasing availability of services, telehealth enables the delivery of care in the least restrictive environment, increases participation of family members in the clinical process, and increases efficiency in delivering services, particularly for itinerant clinicians.[4–8]

TELEHEALTH IN SPEECH-LANGUAGE PATHOLOGY

SLPs have documented the use of telehealth since the 1970s. Early applications and investigations in the use of telecommunication technologies focused on diagnosing and supplementing in-person treatment of neurogenic communication disorders in Veterans' Administration and Mayo Clinic facilities.[9–11] More recently, significant research in the area of telehealth in speech-language pathology has been conducted in Australia, where distances and limited access to SLPs make telehealth a desirable alternative to face-to-face services.[12–20]

ASHA, the professional, scientific, and credentialing association for more than 145,000 SLPs, audiologists, and speech, language, and hearing scientists, has supported the appropriate use of telehealth for over a decade. ASHA developed official policy documents on telepractice (note: telepractice is ASHA's preferred term because it includes applications by SLPs in schools as well as in health care settings) in 2005 and 2010.[21–24] ASHA's position statement affirms that telepractice is an appropriate model of service delivery for the profession of speech-language pathology to "...overcome barriers of access to services caused by distance, unavailability of specialists and/or subspecialists, and impaired mobility."[21] The position statement further stipulates that "...the quality of services must be equivalent to face-to-face."[21] ASHA's 2010 professional issues document describes additional factors contributing to the quality of service, including patient selection, matching appropriate technology to the service being provided, clinician training and competency, and use of patient outcomes and patient and clinician satisfaction measures.[24] Further, the critical importance of having institution-wide training and support is emphasized. Other organizations recognizing the relevance of telepractice for speech-language pathology include professional SLP associations in Canada that have also developed official documents, and the American Telemedicine Association, which has a Special Interest Group for Telerehabilitation.

SLPs have used synchronous interactive video teleconferencing (VTC) to provide services for speech, language, cognitive-communication, voice, and swallowing disorders comparable with those provided in person.[9,12,15,16,25–34] Asynchronous applications have been used as an adjunct to supplement services delivered in person, or to review and validate information observed and recorded during synchronous telepractice/telehealth encounters.[12–20,32]

DEVELOPING TELEHEALTH APPLICATIONS FOR VOICE AND SWALLOWING DISORDERS

It is estimated that voice disorders affect as much as 10% of the United States population and are more prevalent in professional voice users who depend on their voice for work, such as teachers.[35] SLPs and otolaryngologists evaluate patients with voice complaints, and recommend treatment. Voice therapy provided by certified SLPs is effective in addressing behavioral issues contributing to hoarseness.[35,36]

Approximately 10 million Americans with swallowing difficulties are evaluated each year.[37] SLPs perform clinical bedside and/or instrumental assessments such as videofluoroscopy or fiberoptic endoscopy, which are highly sensitive in analyzing the functional swallow and guiding appropriate management.[38,39] Treatment approaches improve nutritional status and hydration, and reduce morbidity from pneumonia.[37]

The telehealth model is suitable for treating voice disorders because of the frequency and intensity of follow-up, with multiple visits for patients who typically do not require acute medical care during the course of rehabilitation. The prevalence of swallowing disorders increases with age and poses particular problems in older patients, including the potential of compromising nutritional status or increasing the risk of aspiration pneumonia, and negatively affecting quality of life. The convenience of receiving specialty services in the home or local community is particularly relevant for the elderly population for whom complex health issues, transportation, or mobility may pose access challenges.

Peripheral devices to support speech-language pathology applications for voice and swallowing include digital audio and video recording devices for a wide range of functions; digital otoscopes for oral mechanism examination; digital fluoroscopes for modified barium swallow studies; fiberoptic video endoscopes to visualize the larynx for fiberoptic endoscopic evaluation of swallow, phonoscopic assessment, or biofeedback training; document cameras to present stimulus materials during evaluation and treatment; pan-tilt-zoom features on cameras for close-up assessment of features or finer movements (eg, check status of tracheoesophageal voice prosthesis, provide instruction on abdominal breath support for voice); and auxiliary video input equipment for computer interfacing.

Procedures that require direct physical contact with the patient are contraindicated for the remote management of voice and swallowing disorders via telehealth. For example, laryngeal palpation is not an option for assessing swallowing dysfunction, and digital laryngeal manipulation and manual circumlaryngeal techniques are not options for assessing musculoskeletal tension or treating muscle tension dysphonia. High bandwidth is typically required to ensure adequate audio and video quality to support clinical decision making during assessment, and for interactive clinical procedures that require immediate and accurate feedback such as to support the establishment of target behaviors during treatment.

Different models of service delivery may be used concomitantly and at different phases of intervention as required for appropriate management. For example, because the quality of video images is critical for visual-perceptual assessment of swallowing or phonoscopic evaluation of vocal function, peripheral devices can be used to capture higher-resolution video data for transmission in the store-and-forward mode to supplement information available during a synchronous consultation, or for review at a later time. Similarly, peripheral devices may be used to obtain higher-fidelity audio data, because the quality of audio samples is critical for auditory-perceptual assessment of voice disorders. During treatment, either in-person or synchronous interaction may be required to establish target behaviors while generalization and maintenance may be achieved with asynchronous follow-up. Audio and video samples may be recorded during real-time guided practice with the clinician, and used as models for home practice. The patient can then record subsequent practice sessions to forward to the clinician for review. Real-time therapy interactions may also be supplemented with electronic mail communication between sessions.

Holtel and Burgess[40] conceptualized a remote Web-based monitoring system using software and peripheral devices including external microphones and headsets to record and assess performance on vocal exercises prescribed during in-person or VTC sessions. Through remote assessment of the patient's status, the clinician can determine (1) the need for a follow-up visit to provide additional instruction or reinforcement, (2) indicators to advance the patient's course of vocal rehabilitation, and (3) readiness for discharge from treatment. Compliance with a vocal health or vocal abuse reduction program could also be monitored remotely.

REMOTE MANAGEMENT OF VOICE DISORDERS

Empirical studies by SLPs support the use of telehealth to diagnose and treat voice disorders remotely. Duffy and colleagues[9] conducted telemedicine consultations at Mayo Clinic facilities between 1987 and 1994. In a review of 150 consultations, 82 patients were diagnosed with voice disorders including spasmodic dysphonia, voice tremor, psychogenic dysphonia, and musculoskeletal tension dysphonia. Otolaryngologic intervention was recommended for 50 patients. The investigators concluded that telemedicine represents a viable alternative to face-to-face consultation when distance precludes timely and cost-effective service, or when specialists are unavailable for speech and language problems that are difficult to diagnose or manage.

Spurred by the aging of the population, extensive rural areas, and difficulty accessing SLPs in Australia, Theodoros and colleagues[15] at the University of Queensland have conducted numerous studies and case reports examining the efficacy and effectiveness of assessment and treatment via telehealth. Their results demonstrate comparable outcomes between in-person and telehealth services for dysarthria, post-laryngectomy, and voice disorders.[17,20,41]

Constantinescu and colleagues[20] investigated the validity and reliability of a telerehabilitation application for assessing the speech and voice disorder associated with Parkinson disease (PD). In simultaneous online and face-to-face environments,

61 participants with PD and hypokinetic dysarthria were evaluated on perceptual measures of voice and oromotor function, articulatory precision, speech intelligibility, and acoustic measures of vocal sound pressure level, phonation time, and pitch range. A personal computer-based videoconferencing system with store-and forward capabilities was used to conduct the online assessments over a 128-Kbps Internet connection. The investigators reported comparable levels of agreement between the two environments for the majority of parameters, and concluded that online assessment of speech and voice in PD appears to be valid and reliable.

In 2003, Mashima and colleagues[30] at Tripler Army Medical Center, Hawaii followed a stepwise process described by research team members Burgess and colleagues[42] in developing and deploying a telehealth vocal rehabilitation protocol as part of a comprehensive telemedicine otolaryngology-head and neck surgery service including audiology and speech pathology. An in-house proof-of-concept study with 51 participants demonstrated no significant differences in auditory-perceptual, acoustic, patient satisfaction, and fiberoptic laryngoscopy outcome ratings between the control (in-person delivery) and experimental (telehealth delivery) groups. Participants in both groups showed positive changes on all 4 outcome measures after completing the vocal rehabilitation protocol. Preliminary data from deployment of remote VTC units to a satellite clinic in rural Oahu and a military hospital in Japan support telehealth as a viable and effective method of service delivery with positive outcomes, including clinician satisfaction with technology used to perform clinical procedures and patient reports of comfort with the technology.[43] Tandberg 880 VTC systems connected via Integrated Services Digital Network (ISDN) lines with 384 Kbps bandwidth were used. Software interfaced with the VTC system and a desktop computer at each site provided the capability to record and analyze voice samples. Laryngeal examinations were performed with a digital videostroboscopy system. Data files of voice samples and laryngeal images were captured, saved, stored, downloaded, and viewed remotely (**Fig. 1**).

Lee Silverman Voice Treatment

The Lee Silverman Voice Treatment (LSVT) LOUD program is a clinical protocol for improving voice and speech in individuals with PD that has been validated by research.[44–48] This intensive program requires therapy 4 times a week for 4 weeks (16 sessions in 1 month) and is delivered by clinicians who are trained and certified by the LSVT Foundation. Barriers that may preclude patients' participation in this treatment include the availability of certified LSVT LOUD clinicians particularly in rural communities, the feasibility of the intense dosage (ie, frequency of therapy sessions), and accessibility issues associated with mobility challenges in individuals with PD that may also require time away from work for a family member or caregiver to provide assistance with attendance. To address these issues and to increase the frequency of long-term follow-up, the LSVT LOUD is now delivered via webcam in patients' homes, offices, senior centers, and nursing home facilities.[49] Specialized training and certification are required for clinicians to deliver LSVT LOUD by telehealth (LSVT eLOUD) to maintain fidelity of the evidence-based program and ensure treatment outcomes comparable with in-person delivery.

Two investigations were independently conducted on the remote delivery of the LSVT. In 2006, Theodoros and colleagues[15] in Australia investigated the feasibility and effectiveness of administering the LSVT at a distance with a 128-Kbps Internet link. Ten participants diagnosed with PD and hypokinetic dysarthria were treated online with the LSVT. The telerehabilitation system used two webcams at the patient's site that were remotely controlled by the clinician's computer with a store-and-forward

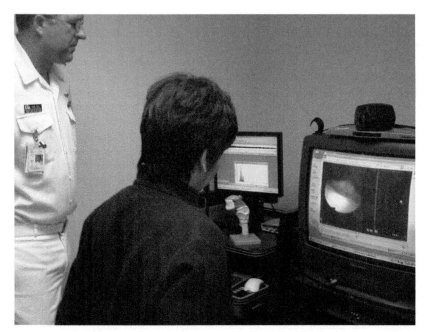

Fig. 1. Joint consultation conducted remotely, with the otolaryngologist diagnosing laryngeal pathology as it affects voice, and the speech-language pathologist assessing voice production and vocal function. The consultation used video teleconferencing (VTC) technology for interactive discussion in real time, and store-and-forward technology to review the prerecorded voice sample and laryngeal examination captured at the remote site. Replay of the voice sample via voice analysis software provided auditory-perceptual and acoustic data while the video endoscopic examination was displayed on the VTC monitor.

component to capture high-quality audio and video recordings for assessment and treatment purposes. The system's speech processor in combination with a headset microphone worn by the patient delivered continuous real-time sound pressure level and pitch data to the clinician. A text transfer application enabled printed treatment materials to be sent by the clinician to the patient's computer. Comparisons of pretreatment and posttreatment results indicated significant increases in sound pressure level and mean pitch range, and significant improvements in perceptual ratings of degree of breathiness, loudness level, and pitch and loudness variability. Although not significantly different from pretreatment ratings, improvement in hoarseness, speech intelligibility, and articulatory precision were identified posttreatment. A majority of participants provided positive feedback regarding the online delivery of therapy; however, some respondents indicated that audio and visual quality were less than adequate with the low-speed bandwidth connection, particularly when degraded during periods of heavy competing Internet traffic.

In 2008, Tindall and colleagues[50] in Kentucky compared the outcomes of LSVT delivered in patients' homes via videophones (Televyou TV 500SP) with published data of the treatment delivered in person. The investigators concluded that treatment delivered via videophone was as effective as in-person treatment based on comparisons of change in decibel levels on prolonged vowel, reading passage, and picture description tasks. Frequency measures or data on pitch range were not reported in this study. Results of a patient satisfaction questionnaire indicated that participants were highly satisfied with videophones as a means of receiving health care services.

Estimated savings in time and cost associated with travel to and from therapy sessions were included in the analyses.

Head and Neck Oncology

SLPs participating in head and neck cancer rehabilitation have used telehealth to improve patient access to subspecialty services that may not be available in rural communities. Professional and peer support are important in adjusting to the effects of the disease and sequelae on communication, eating, and swallowing function that affect quality of life. The potential for social as well as physical isolation is significant. In 2005, Myers[51] reported the use of telehealth VTC technology to provide speech-language pathology services to patients living in remote communities in Manitoba, Canada. Rehabilitation included voice restoration with esophageal and artificial larynx speech; treatment of persistent dysphagia, xerostomia, and dysphonia following chemoradiotherapy; management of premature leakage of a tracheoesophageal voice prosthesis with remote guidance for removal and reinsertion of a new prosthesis; and ongoing education, support, and counseling of patient, family, community members, and health care providers on anatomic, physiologic, and psychosocial consequences of laryngectomy (eg, stoma care, resuscitation of total neck breathers, enhancing communicative exchanges). A social worker and a well-rehabilitated laryngectomee visitor participated in treatment to provide spousal counseling and peer support, and an SLP at the remote site attended sessions to increase her knowledge of postlaryngectomy speech rehabilitation techniques. Technology requirements included a zoom camera feature and good lighting for close-up view to assess status of the stoma, tracheoesophageal voice prosthesis, skin, and mucosa; capability to capture and transfer high-resolution video and still images; and good audio signal to optimize comprehensibility of compromised speech intelligibility. Availability of technical support, nursing assistance, and professional personnel for direct consultation at the remote site as needed was advised.

In 2007, Ward and colleagues[17] compared simultaneous online and in-person assessments with 20 laryngectomees conducted in separate rooms within the same hospital in Australia to validate an Internet-based videoconferencing telerehabilitation system. Assessments were conducted at a bandwidth of 128 Kbps. In addition to enabling the online SLP and patient to view each other throughout the session and communicate via headset microphones, the system also allowed data sharing and captured high-quality audio and video recordings independent of the videoconferencing tools. Results indicated an 80% or higher agreement between the online and in-person clinician for all variables associated with oromotor function, swallowing status, and communication ability. However, inadequate lighting and inability to remotely control zoom/focus of the webcams did not allow adequate visualization of the stoma for clinical decision making when assessing leakage, or fit of a tracheoesophageal voice prosthesis. Online clinicians reported reduced satisfaction with the level of service available via the system and low satisfaction with visual quality, despite high ratings for ease of use and potential for telehealth as a service delivery method. All patients indicated a high level of satisfaction with the usability of the system and quality of services received.

REMOTE MANAGEMENT OF SWALLOWING DISORDERS

There are few published reports of telehealth applications in the area of dysphagia. Three articles describe remote videofluoroscopic examination of oral/pharyngeal swallowing function. In 2002 at the University of Illinois, Urbana-Champaign, Perlman and Witthawaskul[32] developed an Internet-based system that allowed a swallowing specialist to direct a videofluorosocopic study remotely by viewing synchronous video transmission of swallowing images in near real time captured from a fluoroscope at the patient's location. In addition to the transmission-optimized data, full-resolution data were stored for transmission to the specialist at the completion of the evaluation for replay and analysis, including manipulation of the video in real time, frame by frame, at variable speeds, and resizing of images as needed.

In a project funded by a grant from the Office for the Advancement of Telehealth, in 2006 Georges and colleagues[52] used a digital videofluoroscope attached to a Polycom F/X VTC system to capture and transmit images at a rural site in Kansas for consultation with swallowing specialists at the University of Kansas Hospital. Services were well received, and clinicians felt comfortable with the technology. Reported benefits of this telehealth initiative included increased timeliness for modified barium swallow studies, decreased travel and wait time for patients at rural sites, enhanced patient follow-up through prompt discussion of results and recommendations, and opportunity for professional growth and skill development for clinicians at the remote site through interactions with colleagues at the academic medical center.

Malandraki and colleagues[53] conducted a prospective cohort study involving 32 patients to compare fluoroscopic swallowing assessments conducted on-site and via telehealth. The telehealth configuration was described previously by Perlman and Witthawaskul,[32] which consisted of transmitting images from the fluoroscope to the on-site computer and relaying them via broadband Internet connection in real time to the computer at the remote location. A webcam and telephone allowed the off-site clinician to observe the patient and to communicate directly with the patient and staff.

Three variables from the assessments were compared: subjective severity ratings, scores on a penetration-aspiration scale, and agreement in treatment recommendations. The investigators reported good overall agreement for the variables, and concluded that remote assessment offers a promising means of providing swallowing assessments in areas where SLPs with swallowing expertise are unavailable. The primary challenges noted by the investigators included a 1- to 2-second delay during online transmission, and variable quality of the images attributed to excessive Internet traffic, connectivity issues, or other equipment problems. The investigators recommended further testing of their protocol and more studies of short- and long-term outcomes of patients whose swallowing is assessed remotely.

PROFESSIONAL ISSUES IN TELEHEALTH FOR SLPs

While the research to date and interest in telehealth support continues to grow, major barriers to the expansion of telehealth by SLPs are licensure and reimbursement. At present, state licensure laws that address telehealth require SLPs to hold a full license in the state where the patient resides, and in their own state. ASHA has suggested the use of a limited license for telehealth to mitigate this burden.[24]

Telemedicine legislation passed by Congress in 1997 and 2000 designated eligible providers and locations for the delivery of telehealth services that would be reimbursed by Medicare. The list of eligible practitioners does not include SLPs (or audiologists). The lack of Medicare coverage for telehealth services under Part B of the Medicare benefit constrains the development of speech-language pathology services within the United States health care system, leaving the military, Veterans' Administration, or inpatient or home health as the only venues (besides schools, where telehealth is provided by SLPs on a contract basis) that deliver speech-language pathology telehealth services apart from research activities.

However, some states are actively expanding access to telehealth through the development of state telehealth networks and broader reimbursement opportunities. Some state Medicaid programs have designated Current Procedural Terminology codes that may be reimbursed when billed with a telehealth modifier. In addition, approximately 12 states have passed legislation mandating that services covered by private health insurance must also be reimbursed if delivered via telehealth.

FUTURE DIRECTIONS IN REMOTE MANAGEMENT OF VOICE AND SWALLOWING DISORDERS

Additional research is needed to investigate clinical and operational aspects of remote management of voice and swallowing disorders. Outcome measures including clinical effectiveness and clinician and patient satisfaction have been positive in the limited studies available, with the general exception of degraded quality of audio and video signals at low bandwidth transmission (eg, 128 Kbps). This assessment is consistent with a review conducted by Jarvis-Selinger and colleagues[54] in 2008 of 225 articles focused on videoconferencing in clinical contexts including speech-language pathology. These investigators concluded that a minimum bandwidth of 384 Kbps was needed in most applications to establish adequate audio and visual clarity. In addition to technological requirements to support diagnostic protocols and intervention procedures, future research should continue to investigate clinical efficacy and effectiveness, patient and clinician satisfaction, determination of patient candidacy for telehealth, cost-benefit analyses, and practical implementation issues such as scheduling, workflow, and organizational readiness.[24]

SUMMARY

Telehealth or telepractice in speech-language pathology has significant potential to address personnel shortages, unavailability of subspecialists, and barriers in accessing services. Evaluative data are needed to establish evidence-based guidelines and minimal technical requirements to support clinical decision-making for accurate diagnoses and effective treatment comparable to in-person delivery. Additional studies are needed to advance the remote management of voice and swallowing disorders that thus far seems promising, particularly with the ongoing evolution of technological innovations. In addition to research, legislative advocacy is needed to recognize telehealth as a reimbursable service.

ACKNOWLEDGMENTS

The authors thank Dr Michael Holtel, Ms Julia Notarianni, Dr Mark Syms, Mr Greg Suenaga, Mr Neil Sakauye, Mr Sean Wong, Dr Douglas Miller, Dr Lawrence Burgess, Dr Joseph Sniezek, Dr Reese Omizo, Dr Dimitry Goufman, Dr Deborah Birkmire-Peters, Dr Les Peters, and Dr Stan Saiki.

REFERENCES

1. Bureau of Labor Statistics, U.S. Department of Labor. Occupational outlook handbook, 2010-11 edition, speech-language pathologists. Available at: http://www.bls.gov/oco/ocos099.htm#projections_data. Accessed April 30, 2010.
2. American Speech-Language-Hearing Association. 2009 SLP health care survey summary report: number and type of responses. Rockville (MD): American Speech-Language-Hearing Association; 2009.

3. American Speech-Language-Hearing Association. 2005 SLP health care survey summary report: frequency report. Rockville (MD): American Speech-Language-Hearing Association; 2005.

4. Brady A. Moving toward the future: providing speech-language pathology services via telehealth. Home Healthc Nurse 2007;25:240–4.

5. Brennan D. Telemedicine for speech-language pathology: history, challenges, and opportunities. Paper presented at the Institute of Rural Health, Idaho State University; 2006.

6. Brown JE, Carpenedo DJ. Managing urban speech therapy caseloads successfully by using telehealth. Caring 2006;25:54–6.

7. Carpenedo DJ. Telepractice in the city: the story of the visiting nurse service of New York home care. ASHA Lead 2006;11:10–1.

8. Mashima PA, Birkmire-Peters DP, Holtel MR, et al. Telehealth applications in speech-language pathology. J Healthc Inf Manag 1999;13(4):71–8.

9. Duffy JR, Werven GW, Aronson AE. Telemedicine and the diagnosis of speech and language disorders. Mayo Clin Proc 1997;72:1116–22.

10. Vaughn GR. Tele-communicology: health-care delivery system for persons with communication disorders. ASHA 1976;18(1):13–7.

11. Wertz RT, Dronkers NF, Bernstein-Ellis E, et al. Potential of telephonic and television technology for appraising and diagnosing neurogenic communication disorders in remote settings. Aphasiology 1992;6:195–202.

12. Hill AJ, Theodoros DG, Russell TG, et al. An internet-based telerehabilitation system for the assessment of motor speech disorders: a pilot study. Am J Speech Lang Pathol 2006;15:45–56.

13. O'Brian S, Packman A, Onslow M. Telehealth delivery of the Camperdown Program for adults who stutter: a phase I trial. J Speech Lang Hear Res 2008; 51:184–95.

14. Theodoros D, Hill A, Russell T, et al. Assessing acquired language disorders in adults via the Internet. Telemed J E Health 2008;14(6):552–9.

15. Theodoros DG, Constantinescu G, Russell TG, et al. Treating the speech disorder in Parkinson's disease online. J Telemed Telecare 2006;12(Suppl 3):S3:88–91.

16. Waite MC, Cahill LM, Theodoros DG, et al. A pilot study of online assessment of childhood speech disorders. J Telemed Telecare 2006;12(Suppl 3):S3:92–4.

17. Ward L, White J, Russell T, et al. Assessment of communication and swallowing function post laryngectomy: a telerehabilitation trial. J Telemed Telecare 2007; 13(Suppl 3):S3:88–91.

18. Wilson L, Onslow M, Lincoln M. Telehealth adaptation of the Lidcombe Program of early stuttering intervention: five case studies. Am J Speech Lang Pathol 2004; 13:81–93.

19. Hill AJ, Theodoros D, Russell T, et al. Using telerehabilitation to assess apraxia of speech in adults. Int J Lang Commun Disord 2009;44(5):731–47.

20. Constantinescu G, Theodoros D, Russell T, et al. Assessing disordered speech and voice in Parkinson's disease: a telerehabilitation application. Int J Lang Commun Disord 2010;45(6):630–44.

21. American Speech-Language-Hearing Association. Speech-language pathologists providing clinical services via telepractice: [Position Statement], 2005. Available at: www.asha.org/policy. Accessed April 30, 2010.

22. American Speech-Language-Hearing Association. Speech-language pathologists providing clinical services via telepractice [Technical Report], 2005. Available at: www.asha.org/policy. Accessed April 30, 2010.

23. American Speech-Language-Hearing Association. Knowledge and skills needed by speech-language pathologists providing clinical services via telepractice [Knowledge and Skills], 2005. Available at: www.asha.org/policy. Accessed April 30, 2010.
24. American-Speech-Language-Hearing Association. Professional issues in telepractice for speech-language pathologists [Professional Issues], 2010. Available at: www.asha.org/policy. Accessed April 30, 2010.
25. Brennan DM, Georgeadis AC, Baron CR, et al. The effect of videoconference-based telerehabilitation on story retelling performance by brain-injured subjects and its implications for remote speech-language therapy. Telemed J E Health 2004;10:147–54.
26. Georgeadis AC, Brennan DM, Barker LM, et al. Telerehabilitation and its effect on storytelling by adults with neurogenic disorders. Aphasiology 2004;18: 639–52.
27. Grogan-Johnson S, Alvares RL, Rowan L, et al. A pilot study comparing the effectiveness of speech-language therapy provided by telepractice. J Telemed Telecare 2010;16:134–9.
28. Kully D. Telehealth in speech-language pathology: applications to the treatment of stuttering. J Telemed Telecare 2000;6(2):39–41.
29. McCullough A. Viability and effectiveness of teletherapy for pre-school children with special needs. Int J Lang Commun Disord 2001;36(Suppl):321–6.
30. Mashima PA, Birkmire-Peters DP, Syms MJ, et al. Telehealth: voice therapy using telecommunications technology. Am J Speech Lang Pathol 2003;12:432–9.
31. Palsbo SE. Equivalence of functional communication assessment in speech pathology using videoteleconferencing. J Telemed Telecare 2007;13:40–3.
32. Perlman AL, Witthawaskul W. Real-time remote telefluoroscopic assessment of patients with dysphagia. Dysphagia 2002;17:162–7.
33. Rose DA, Furner S, Hall A, et al. Videoconferencing for speech and language therapy in schools. BT Technol J 2000;18:101–4.
34. Sicotte C, Lehoux P, Fortier-Blanc J, et al. Feasibility and outcome evaluation of a telemedicine application in speech-language pathology. J Telemed Telecare 2003;9:253–8.
35. American Speech-Language-Hearing Association. Treatment efficacy summary: laryngeal-based voice disorders. 2008. Available at: http://www.asha.org/uploadedFiles/public/TreatmentEfficacySummaries2008.pdf. Accessed April 30, 2010.
36. Schwartz SR, Cohen SM, Dailey SH, et al. Clinical practice guideline: hoarseness (dysphonia). Otolaryngol Head Neck Surg 2009;141:S1–31.
37. American Speech-Language-Hearing Association. Communication facts: special populations: dysphagia—2008 edition. Available at: http://www.asha.org/research/reports/dysphagia.htm. Accessed April 30, 2010.
38. American Speech-Language-Hearing Association. Guidelines for speech-language pathologists performing videofluoroscopic swallowing studies [Guidelines], 2004. Available at: www.asha.org/policy. Accessed May 4, 2010.
39. American Speech-Language-Hearing Association. The role of the speech-language pathologist in the performance and interpretation of endoscopic evaluation of swallowing [Position Statement], 2005. Available at: www.asha.org/policy. Accessed May 4, 2010.
40. Holtel MR, Burgess LP. Telemedicine in otolaryngology. Otolaryngol Clin North Am 2002;35:1263–81.

41. Hill AJ, Theodoros DG, Russell TG, et al. The redesign and re-evaluation of an internet-based telerehabilitation system for the assessment of dysarthria in adults. Telemed J E Health 2009;15(9):840–50.

42. Burgess LP, Holtel MR, Syms MJ, et al. Overview of telemedicine applications for otolaryngology. Laryngoscope 1999;109:1433–7.

43. Mashima PA, Holtel MR. Telepractice brings voice treatment from Hawaii to Japan. ASHA Lead 2005;10:20–1, 45.

44. Spielman J, Ramig LO, Mahler L, et al. Effects of an extended version of the Lee Silverman voice treatment on voice and speech in Parkinson's disease. Am J Speech Lang Pathol 2007;16:95–107.

45. Fox CM, Ramig LO, Ciucci MR, et al. The science and practice of LSVT/LOUD: neural plasticity—principled approach to treating individuals with Parkinson disease and other neurological disorders. Semin Speech Lang 2006;27(4): 283–99.

46. Baumgartner CA, Sapir S, Ramig LO. Voice quality changes following phonatory-respiratory effort treatment (LSVT) versus respiratory effort treatment for individuals with Parkinson disease. J Voice 2001;15(1):105–14.

47. Ramig LO, Countryman S, Thompson LL, et al. Comparison of two forms of intensive speech treatment for Parkinson's disease. J Speech Hear Res 1995;38(6): 1232–51.

48. Constantinescu GA, Theodoros DG, Russell TG, et al. Home-based speech treatment for Parkinson's disease delivered remotely: a case report. J Telemed Telecare 2010;16(2):100–4.

49. "What is LSVT eLOUD?" LSVT Global brochure found at. Available at: http://www.lsvtglobal.com/index.php?action=what-is-eloud. Accessed April 17, 2010.

50. Tindall LR, Huebner RA, Stemple JC, et al. Videophone-delivered voice therapy: a comparative analysis of outcomes to traditional delivery for adults with Parkinson's disease. Telemed J E Health 2008;14(10):1070–7.

51. Myers C. Telehealth applications in head and neck oncology. Revue d'orthophonie et d'audiologie 2005;29(3):125–9.

52. Georges J, Potter K, Belz N. Telepractice program for dysphagia: urban and rural perspectives from Kansas. ASHA Lead 2006;11:12.

53. Malandraki GA, McCullough G, He X, et al. Teledynamic evaluation of oropharyngeal swallowing. J Speech Lang Hear Res, in press.

54. Jarvis-Selinger S, Chan E, Payne R, et al. Clinical telehealth across the disciplines: lessons learned. Telemed J E Health 2008;14:720–5.

Robotics and Telesurgery in Otolaryngology

Jason G. Newman, MD[a],*, Ronald B. Kuppersmith, MD, MBA[b],
Bert W. O'Malley Jr, MD[c]

KEYWORDS

- Robotic surgery • Telesurgery • TORS
- Robotic thyroid surgery • Robotic skull base surgery
- Robotic otolaryngology • Robotic head and neck surgery

Robotic technology has been widely used in many nonmedical industries for more than 50 years. However, medical applications in robotics became commonly available only recently. In 1985, the first robotic-assisted procedure was performed, used to accurately localize neurosurgical biopsies. The same device (Puma 560) was then used to perform transurethral biopsies of the prostate. However, despite these advances, the interest in robotics in medicine was still weak. In 1992, the U.S. Food and Drug Administration (FDA) approved the first medical use of a robot. At about the same time, the National Aeronautics and Space Administration and the Department of Defense, recognizing that having a surgeon available on the front lines attending to wounded soldiers during the "golden hour" of trauma would be difficult, began to explore the concept of telepresence battlefield surgery. In theory, a robotic setup could be deployed into frontline battlefield zones, and surgery could be performed remotely on an injured soldier, by a team operating from a safe zone. The Department of Defense, through the Defense Advanced Research Projects Agency, invested significant time and money into this application, which helped boost the general interest in robotics in medicine. This influx of funding and scientific interest finally created enough momentum that the technology began to reach into routine nonmilitary medical applications. This process accelerated the creation of the first commercially available robotic systems, the AESOP (Computer Motion of Santa

No funding support was received for the publication of this article.
Jason G. Newman has received support from Intuitive Surgical for proctoring of surgical cases.
[a] Department of Otorhinolaryngology-Head and Neck Surgery, The University of Pennsylvania Health System, 811 Spruce Street, Philadelphia, PA 19107, USA
[b] 1730 Birmingham Drive, College Station, TX 77845, USA
[c] Department of Otorhinolaryngology-Head and Neck Surgery, The University of Pennsylvania Health System, 3400 Spruce Street-5 Ravdin, Philadelphia, PA 19104, USA
* Corresponding author.
E-mail address: Jason.newman@uphs.upenn.edu

Otolaryngol Clin N Am 44 (2011) 1317–1331
doi:10.1016/j.otc.2011.08.008
0030-6665/11/$ – see front matter © 2011 Elsevier Inc. All rights reserved.

Barbara, CA, USA) and the da Vinci (Intuitive Surgical, Sunnyvale, CA, USA) systems. Variations of these are still commercially in use today.

The basic concept of telepresence on the battlefield is the premise for the evolving concept of telesurgery, whereby the surgeon performing the operation is not in the same location (or operating room area) as the patient. In general, telesurgery infers a significant distance between the patient and the surgeon, whether this be across town or between states or countries. A major advance of telesurgery is that it brings the expert surgeon to the patient and obviates the need for the patient to travel to the surgeon. This concept of telesurgery, and telemedicine overall, has both national and world health advantages, wherein high-level care could theoretically be provided to underserved areas and populations. Although it seems natural to expand classic robotic surgery as performed today into routine telesurgery, many more complexities exist with respect to the requirements for advanced communications technology and extreme high-speed and dedicated data connections. The feasibility of intercontinental robotic telesurgery was established in 2001 by surgeons in New York performing a cholecystectomy on a patient in Paris. The present hurdles in information management and data transfer over the Internet or dedicated communication portals must be overcome to make telesurgery a reality.

In otolaryngology-head and neck surgery, the primary robotic system in use is the da Vinci system. It consists of a two major components. The first component is the surgeon console, which is a master control where the primary surgeon sits to manipulate the robotic arms. The second component is the robotic cart, which is manipulated remotely by the operating surgeon. The current technology allows the surgeon to manipulate up to three arms with wristed, interchangeable instruments, and one stereoscopic (three-dimensional image) camera, also manipulated from the surgeon console. The robotic instruments, unlike most endoscopic and laparoscopic instruments, are designed to mimic and even exceed the natural range of movement of the surgeon wrists, giving 7° of freedom (**Fig. 1**A and B). With respect to the high-powered optics, the robotic telescope actually incorporates two separate cameras in the distal tip, offset by 15°, giving a true stereoscopic, three-dimensional, high-definition view of the field (**Fig. 2**). The combination of the wristed movement, distal

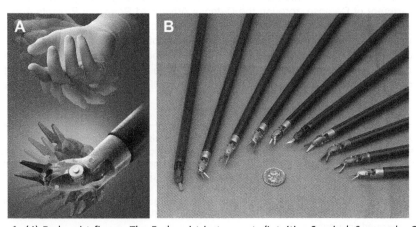

Fig. 1. (*A*) Endowrist figure. The Endowrist instruments (Intuitive Surgical, Sunnyvale, CA, USA) have 6° of freedom, mimicking the surgeon's wrist in the ability to rotate and bend. (*B*) Instruments with dime. An example of the array of instruments available and interchangeable for use with the robotic console. (*Courtesy of* Intuitive Surgical, Inc., Sunnyvale, CA. Copyright © 2011 Intuitive Surgical, Inc., with permission.)

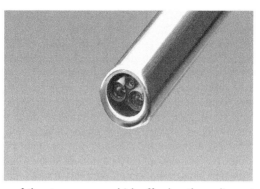

Fig. 2. Close up view of the stereoscope, which affords a three-dimensional view with two separate cameras providing a high-definition view of the surgical field. (*Courtesy of* Intuitive Surgical, Inc., Sunnyvale, CA. Copyright © 2011 Intuitive Surgical, Inc., with permission.)

dexterity, and three-dimensional view are what make this tool well suited for surgery within a confined space (**Fig. 3**).

In the field of otolaryngology–head and neck surgery, robotics has only a brief history. Initial reports in the literature from the early 2000s described the use of the da Vinci robotic system to help minimize incisions in the neck.[1,2] The first reported case in a live patient was the excision of a benign vallecular cyst.[3]

Shortly thereafter, Weinstein and colleagues[4] described the first transoral robotic surgery (TORS). The concept was adapted from the evolving use of robotics in the field of urology and cardiac surgery. If the robotic instruments could be placed through small incisions to access the heart or prostate, it seemed reasonable to explore their use in the pharynx and larynx. Furthermore, the trend toward less-invasive and endoscopic procedures in otolaryngology-head and neck surgery led many physicians to explore alternative means of approaching well-established open surgical techniques. Much like endoscopic or laparoscopic surgery, robotic surgery allows surgeons to

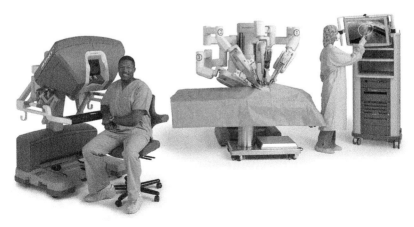

Fig. 3. The three components of the da Vinci Si robot include the surgeon console, the patient cart, and the vision cart. (*Courtesy of* Intuitive Surgical, Inc., Sunnyvale, CA. Copyright © 2011 Intuitive Surgical, Inc., with permission.)

place instruments into small openings or orifices, allowing distal dexterity that would otherwise be difficult to achieve without large incisions.

Much of the early work in robotics came from the fields of cardiac and urologic surgery.[5,6] In both of these fields, robotic surgery has now become somewhat routine. In fact, in 2009, more than 85% of men treated surgically for prostate cancer had the surgery performed with robotic assistance. On the heels of the success of robotics in these specialties, other fields of surgical medicine have adopted the use of robotics. Gynecology and bariatric surgery have created several applications for robotic surgery.[7,8] Other subspecialties are also beginning to consider robotic applications.

The initial preclinical experiments establishing the premise of transoral robotic surgery were performed by O'Malley and Hockstein at the University of Pennsylvania.[4,9] These early experiments were conducted on human airway mannequins. Building on these original studies, Hockstein and colleagues[10–12] established a true preclinical research program with both cadaver and live canine experimental models for developing novel robotic surgical techniques and testing the feasibility of robotic surgery as it applies to the field of otolaryngology–head and neck surgery.

One of the first obstacles to overcome in adapting the robotic instruments to the mouth was the laryngoscope. Conventionally, most laryngoscopes have a narrow inlet, and the configuration and size of the robotic arms cannot work within this space. However, several instruments were available and useful to overcome this problem. The Dingman retractor, Crow Davis retractor, and the FK laryngoscope (Gyrus Ent LLC, Bartlett, TN, USA) were some of the early devices used to gain access to the laryngopharynx and allow adequate mobility of the robotic arms for surgery (**Fig. 4**). Using these retractors, the robotic arms could gain access to the laryngopharynx via the oral cavity. With respect to the cadaver and canine experiments, the original procedures evaluated were vocal cord stripping, partial cordectomy, mucosal flap harvest and inset, tongue base resection, and arytenoidectomy. The authors concluded that this technology may increase the precision of many of these procedures.

After these technical feasibility and discovery studies were completed in cadavers, additional studies were designed and performed to evaluate the safety or to identify risks in using robotic instruments for transoral or head and neck procedures in general. Hemostasis, inadvertent facial and oral injury, and general safety precautions were evaluated. These studies concluded that the safety profile of the robotic-assisted surgical procedures is similar to that of conventional transoral surgery.[10] The combination of technical feasibility and safety established in the preclinical work cleared the way for human trials.

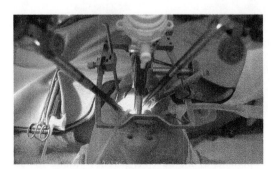

Fig. 4. FK retractor in oral cavity. The FK retractor allows for a wide approach to the laryngopharynx, affording greater range of motion for the robotic arms.

Weinstein and O'Malley[13] established a prospective Institutional Review Board (IRB)–approved human trial at the University of Pennsylvania and conducted the first human experiments for TORS. The original human trials included patients with tonsil, base of tongue, and supraglottic cancers, and a variety of benign tumors and lesions that could be accessed transorally. The trials investigated the safety of the surgery, the optimal instrumentation, and the rate of complications (**Fig. 5**). Results showed that TORS could be performed in a safe and effective manner, with minimal complications.[13,14] After the initial surgical trials, further data were collected to show the appropriateness, safety, and efficacy of this procedure. This compiled data were presented to the FDA and, in December 2009, TORS was approved in the United States to treat benign tumors or lesions and selected T1 and T2 malignant tumors in adults. The use of TORS for larger lesions (T3 and T4) is not currently approved by the FDA and merits more investigation.

The TORS operating room setup involves several steps to dock the robot and ensure adequate exposure of the surgical field:

- Once the patient is intubated with a reinforced tube, the table is turned away from the anesthesia cart to give the robotic patient cart more room to maneuver.
- The appropriate laryngoscope or retractor is placed and suspended.
- The endotracheal tube is sewn in place to retract it out of the surgical field and reduce the chance of inadvertent extubation.
- The robotic console is brought in from a 30° angle from the patient, and the robotic instruments are introduced into the oral cavity.
- The primary surgeon begins at the console, and the bedside surgeon assists by retracting and suctioning at the head of the patient.

OROPHARYNGEAL TORS

Tonsil and base of tongue cancer resections are among the more commonly performed procedures with TORS. Before the advent of TORS, patients with oropharyngeal cancers who were treated surgically often required classic mandibulotomy, tracheostomy, and often free flap or other reconstructions to achieve successful negative-margin surgery. In selected cases, TORS allows these patients the option of completely transoral approach (**Fig. 6**). In the analysis of the first 27 patients

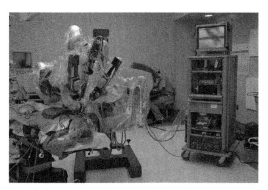

Fig. 5. Demonstration of the room and patient setup for TORS cases. Not shown is the bedside surgical assistant, who is helping with retraction and suctioning, and general monitoring of the patient.

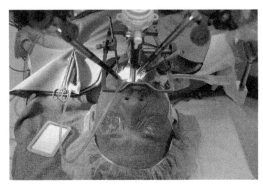

Fig. 6. Oropharynx approach. With the patient in suspension, the combination of the 30° stereoscope and the wristed instruments allow the surgeon to access the base of the tongue for complete visualization and resection of tumor.

undergoing this approach, the results showed a low incidence of morbidity, with no perioperative mortality. In this series, one patient developed a bleed, and another required a tracheostomy.[15]

To be a candidate for TORS for oropharynx cancer, certain patient and tumor characteristics must be met:

- The most obvious is that the tumor must be adequately visualized and exposed for resection.
- Characteristics such as trismus, anterior positioned larynx, large tongue, or morbid obesity often make placement of the pharyngeal retractors impossible.
- During staging laryngoscopy, the appropriate retractors may need to be inserted to determine if the tumor will be amenable to negative-margin resection with TORS techniques.

The following characteristics are also considered contraindications for TORS[15]:

- Unresectability of involved neck nodes
- Mandibular invasion
- Tongue base involvement requiring resection of greater than 50% of the tongue base
- Pharyngeal wall involvement necessitating resection of more than 50% of the posterior pharyngeal wall
- Radiologic confirmation of carotid artery involvement
- Prevertebral fascia fixation of tumor.

After the resection, a decision is made regarding the need for continued intubation. Many patients with tongue base resections benefit from remaining intubated postoperatively, until the edema created by the surgery has a chance to regress. This process often requires approximately 48 hours. In patients who primarily undergo surgery in the region of the tonsil, this is often not necessary.

Neck dissections are almost always necessary in this population, and most studies have advocated delaying this portion of the surgery for 1 to 4 weeks. The rationale is to reduce the chance of orocutaneous fistula, and to reduce the laryngopharyngeal edema related to both the length of the surgery and the instrumentation in the pharynx and neck concomitantly.

LARYNGEAL TORS

Before the introduction of TORS, laser microsurgery for select glottic and supraglottic lesions had established itself as a safe and effective means to manage these tumors. TORS takes advantage of many of the characteristics of laser procedures, and adds several others, making it an excellent alternative to laser resections. In addition to oral access to the larynx, TORS affords the operating surgeon excellent distal control of instrumentation and removal of the line of site issues that can occur with the operating microscope, allowing great dexterity in the resection and management of these tumors (**Fig. 7**).

Much like decision making in oropharynx lesions, choosing appropriate candidates for this surgery is critical. Not only is it important to confirm that the tumor can be adequately resected via this approach but also the operating surgeon must feel that surgery will produce the best functional outcome (relative to nonsurgical approaches).

Not surprisingly, these patients have a slightly higher rate of temporary tracheostomy in the combination of trials performed in the literature. Furthermore, the rate of dysphagia seems slightly higher in patients undergoing laryngeal TORS compared with oropharyngeal TORS.[16]

The instrumentation to perform laryngeal microsurgery is still being designed. Despite the excellent visibility and dexterity of the robotic arms, the lack of fine instrumentation and the limitations imposed by the relatively large robotic arms and camera still pose a challenge for managing many of the tumors below the level of the supraglottis.

Robotic Thyroidectomy

Transaxillary robotic thyroidectomy is another application of robotics in the field of otolaryngology–head and neck surgery. Although this technique evolved from attempts to reduce or eliminate the cervical incisions that have generally been the hallmark of thyroid surgery for more than 100 years, it may ultimately allow surgeons to become facile with endoscopic neck surgery. Although TORS eliminates the incisions related to resection of the primary, many of these patients still require an open neck dissection. Researchers have postulated that mastery of these techniques, initially through thyroid surgery, will ultimately allow head and neck cancer to be managed entirely via an endoscopic approach.[17]

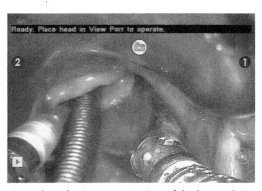

Fig. 7. Robot larynx view. The robotic surgeon's view of the larynx during supraglottic laryngectomy. The ability of the instruments to turn corners eliminates the "line of sight" issues that make laser surgery difficult.

Over the years, thyroidectomy incisions have become smaller in selected patients. The application of endoscopes has allowed for video-assisted thyroid surgery. Several authors described various approaches to the thyroid using incisions hidden from view, including inframammary, areolar, and even transoral approaches to the thyroid gland, typically using carbon dioxide (CO_2) insufflation to maintain a working space. An endoscopic transaxillary approach to this region had been developed both with and without CO_2 insufflation. After a significant experience with the endoscopic approach, robotic technology was applied (**Fig. 8**).

One of the pioneers of the robotic transaxillary approach to the thyroid is Dr Chung at Yonsei hospital in Korea. He has performed and reported on more than 500 robotic thyroid cases, with excellent results.[18] More recently, this surgery gained popularity in the United States, and several studies have been designed to evaluate its feasibility and safety.[19]

Generally, the robotic transaxillary approach to the thyroid involves creating a surgical working space.

- The space is maintained with a retractor instead of insufflation.
- A plane is created from the axilla, over the pectoralis muscle, and the heads of the sternocleidomastoid muscle are separated.
- The strap muscles are retracted anteriorly–anteriorly, allowing access to the lateral aspect of the thyroid bed.
- The robotic instruments are then brought into the field and the thyroid is removed.
- The contralateral lobe is removed through dissecting over the trachea and taking a medial-to-lateral approach to the gland.

The obvious benefit of the robotic approach to the thyroid through the axilla is the lack of a neck incision. In addition, possible added benefits relate to magnified stereoscopic visualization and improved dexterity. These benefits must be shown through comparative trials. Additionally, potential complications that do not typically occur during traditional thyroid surgery must be considered because of the lateral approach, including injury to the carotid artery, jugular vein, and esophagus.

The Role of Robotics in Teaching

Robotics lends itself easily to serving as a teaching tool. Even as an observer of the procedure, the visualization is excellent. With the exception of the stereoscopic

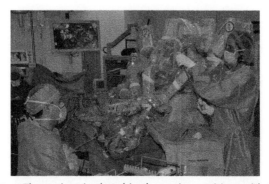

Fig. 8. Thyroid setup. The patient is placed in the supine position, with the arm extended over the head. In this photograph, the patient's head is on the right and the feet are facing the anesthesia team. The arms are introduced at an acute lateral angle to gain access to the thyroid through the axilla.

view, observers are seeing the same field as the surgeon. Additionally, some centers are equipped with three-dimensional observation screens to provide a more realistic view for observers.

Another useful tool that serves as a teaching aid for robotic surgery with the da Vinci robot is the telestration capacity (**Fig. 9**). Although the surgical student sits at the console, the teacher can use one of the real-time monitors to draw and illustrate in a manner that be seen by the physician at the console. This technique allows a hands-on approach by the teacher, even while the student is at the console.

The newest generation of the da Vinci surgical robot (Si) has even more potential as a teaching tool. It has an option for an integrated two-console station (**Fig. 10**). These two consoles allow for two separate surgeons to be involved in a procedure. If it is set up as a teacher–student, the student can perform the surgery and the teacher can direct movements with visible pointers, or can take over control of the robotic arms from the student to show a technique. Although most of these two-surgeon procedures are still being performed with both surgeons in the same operating suite, it is easy to imagine that they could be in separate operating rooms, or even different countries as the technology improves.

To date, limited studies in otolaryngology–head and neck surgery have described the use of long-distance telesurgery for more than experimental investigations. At least one report in the literature has shown the feasibility of telesurgery. This experiment, performed in Zagreb, Croatia, described computer-assisted remote endoscopic surgery.[20]

Limitations of robotics

The authors have adapted instrumentation designed for laparoscopic surgery to use in their procedures in the field of otolaryngology–head and neck surgery. Most of the instruments, which vary in size from 5 to 8 mm in diameter, are still large. As surgeons in this field continue to explore uses for robotics, one would expect that instruments will be designed for the specific surgery. In fact, surgeons at many centers are working to design instruments and even robots that may be more well suited to the anatomic constraints of the head and neck structures.

The inability to "feel" the surgical field (*haptic feedback*) is also a limitation of robotic surgery. Although this same problem exists in endoscopic surgery, it is present to

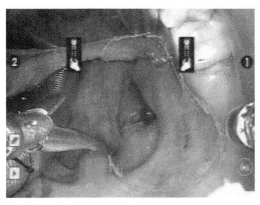

Fig. 9. Telestration with TORS. The nonoperating surgeon can easily draw and illustrate on one of the operative monitors. The operating surgeon can see this overlay on the stereoscopic view.

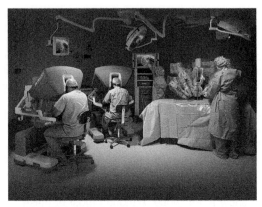

Fig. 10. Two-surgeon setup. With a dual-console setup, two surgeons can be involved in the surgery at the same time. This configuration can be used in a teacher–student setup, or in a primary–assistant setup. (*Courtesy of* Intuitive Surgical, Inc., Sunnyvale, CA. Copyright © 2011 Intuitive Surgical, Inc., with permission.)

a greater degree in robotic surgery, where no connection exists between the instrument and the surgeon's hand. Although several authors have commented that the exceptional optics used by the robot make this issue less concerning, most seem to agree that haptic feedback would be advantageous, especially in areas such as the base of tongue, where the feel of the soft tissue is often what surgeons use to determine how close to the margin of the tumor they are dissecting.

One of the clear advantages of robotic head and neck surgery for cancer is the lack of incision in the treatment of diseases of the laryngopharynx. In light of this, the need for an open neck dissection in many of these patients raises the obvious question of whether this incision can be eliminated. Dr Chung already described a transaxillary modified neck dissection. Whether this procedure will prove safe and effective in the management of lymphadenopathy from head and neck cancers remains to be seen.

The question of cost-effectiveness for these surgical procedures is an important one. Especially in the modern era of medicine, this is an important factor to consider in decision making. No published study has yet addressed this issue in the field of otolaryngology–head and neck surgery. However, this question has been addressed by cost comparisons in other fields.[21–23] The authors of the studies have generally compared the cost of the robotic surgery to the cost of another approach. In general, they have concluded that the surgical cost is higher. The caveat, as mentioned by several of the authors, is that the postoperative course and the rate of complications may be lower. In the articles in which the robotic technique seemed to add no appreciable benefit, the conclusion was that the added cost of the robotic procedure is not justified. In addition, none of the studies compared the cost of the robotic surgery with the cost of chemotherapy and radiation for the same disease.

A significant learning curve is associated with mastering robotic technology and these new surgical approaches. For both TORS and robotic thyroid surgery obtaining appropriate exposure to perform safe surgery is one of the most challenging aspects of these procedures. Surgeons should obtain adequate training to ensure proficiency before performing these procedures. During the informed consent process, patients must be educated about potential risks associated with these new procedures and the limited outcomes data available relative to traditional approaches. Surgeons should also inform patients about their own experience and outcomes with these approaches.

The Future of Robotics in Otolaryngology–Head and Neck Surgery

The technology to perform more complex and targeted robotic procedures continues to evolve. The development of smaller instruments, new surgical approaches, improved laser delivery systems, and procedure-specific devices will increase the potential benefits even further. Single-port, snake-like technology has emerged as an even less-invasive approach for robotic-assisted surgery. Although no clinical systems currently exist, conceptually a single-entry port could allow several arms to emerge, triangulating once inside of the surgical space to perform the surgery.

As new instrumentation becomes available, the application of this technology to other aspects of otolaryngology, including the middle ear, lateral and anterior skull base, and sinus cavities, may come to fruition.

Some initial studies have shown the feasibility of tongue base resection for obstructive sleep apnea. Sleep apnea remains a poorly understood disease affecting between 4% and 10% of the United States population, and more than 70% of patients who are obese. Many procedures have been proposed for its treatment, but most have failed to achieve good long-term results. Surgical resection of the base of the tongue has proven to be challenging. In their prospective human trial, O'Malley and Weinstein[13] established the feasibility and rationale of using TORS for resection of tongue base tumors and limited benign and inflammatory lesions of the tongue. Based on the human trial experience, Vicini and colleagues[24] initiated a study to evaluate the safety and efficacy of TORS for resection of the tongue base for sleep apnea. Preliminary results in a series of 10 patients with obstructive apnea-hypopnea syndrome showed that robotic management of the tongue base is feasible. Long-term results are not yet published, and the role for this procedure as part of comprehensive surgical management of the airway in sleep apnea still must be investigated. Thaler, Weinstein, and O'Malley initiated a prospective IRB-approved human trial investigating TORS for sleep apnea at the University of Pennsylvania in 2009, personal communications.

With respect to the skull base, studies have shown that the techniques were feasible, and that the midline and anterior base of skull could be safely approached with current instrumentation.[25] In 2007, a patient with a high parapharyngeal base of skull tumor underwent successful robotic resection at the University of Pennsylvania by O'Malley and Weinstein.[25] Since then, several techniques have been described to more effectively approach and navigate this area. Cervical-TORS, one of the earliest techniques, involved placing two of the robotic instrument actuators through a percutaneously dilated cervical incision just behind the submandibular gland.[26] This technique allowed visualization and instrumentation at the clivus, sella, sphenoid, and suprasellar anterior fossa (**Figs. 11** and **12**). Another approach, described by Hanna and colleagues,[27] involved performing bilateral Caldwell-Luc type incisions, allowing the robotic actuators to transcend the maxilla, entering the nasal cavity through an enlarged antrotomy. Finally, more recent studies have shown the feasibility of placing all of the instruments transnasally to access the anterior base of skull, sella, and clivus.

Other areas of the cranial base being investigated are the craniocervical junction and atlantoaxial region. Lee and colleagues[28] performed cadaver studies, followed by early clinical trials, which have shown the feasibility of these techniques in helping to approach and visualize this complex region. Currently, clinical trials are underway to study transoral robotic-assisted odontoidectomy. Using the conventional nonrobotic approach, patients having this surgery generally undergo a transoral or transnasal

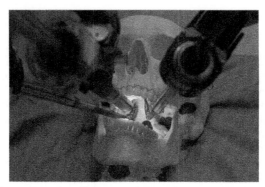

Fig. 11. Skull configuration. The advantage of wristed instrumentation and angled stereo-scope is the ability to perform surgery on the cranial base around the oropharyngeal inlet, as shown on a model.

approach to the odontoid using either a headlight or endoscope. The robotic technique allows for a clear unobstructed stereoscopic view of the entire high cervical spine up to the odontoid (**Fig. 13**). Prevertebral dissection can be safely and accurately performed using the articulated robotic instruments. The patients can then undergo

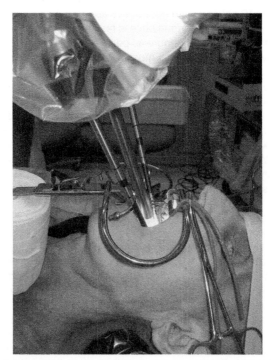

Fig. 12. Cadaver skull base. For the approach to the cranial base, the patient cart is docked at the head of the patient, allowing angled access to the superior portion of the nasal cavity or oropharynx.

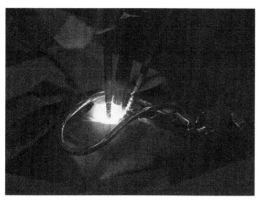

Fig. 13. Patient undergoing the odontoid approach. Using the Crockard retractor (Codman, Raynham, MA, USA), the robotic arms are inserted into the oral cavity, giving the operating surgeon an exceptional view of the posterior pharyngeal wall.

precise prevertebral fascia and mucosa closure to reduce dehiscence and a possible cerebrospinal fluid leak postoperatively (**Fig. 14**). To date, this procedure has been performed in four patients, all successfully.

Applications in the skull base have clarified some of the current limitations of robotic surgery. The lack of bone cutting instruments and drills has limited the use in these arenas. In addition, despite the excellent dexterity and clarity of view, the current instrumentations are still not fine enough to perform the delicate dissections necessary in this region. However, it is already clear that modifications to some of the existing instrumentation will have the potential to drastically affect the ability to perform robotic surgery in this region. Unlike with nonwristed instrumentation, robotic instrumentation has the potential to quickly replace multiple instruments with a single well-designed one.

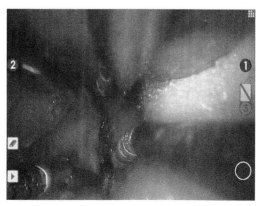

Fig. 14. Odontoid robot view. View of the operating surgeon during robotic posterior pharyngeal wall dissection. Tongue is superior and soft palate is inferior in this view. Note the ability of the electrocautery to curve around the soft palate.

SUMMARY

The history of robotics in the field of otolaryngology–head and neck surgery has been brief. However, great advances have been made within this short period. The technology has gone from preclinical trials to clinical experimentation, to full clinical implementation in less than 10 years. Treatment of a wide range of diseases in the oropharynx and larynx is feasible with TORS, and significant headway is being made with robotic assistance for the neck, thyroid, and base of skull. As the procedures continue to evolve, and the technology continues to improve, robotic surgery is likely to continue to play a larger role in the treatment of diseases of the head and neck.

REFERENCES

1. Gourin CG, Terris DJ. Surgical robotics in otolaryngology: expanding the technology envelope. Curr Opin Otolaryngol Head Neck Surg 2004;12(3):204–8.
2. Haus BM, Kambham N, Le D, et al. Surgical robotic applications in otolaryngology. Laryngoscope 2003;113(7):1139–44.
3. McLeod IK, Melder PC. Da Vinci robot-assisted excision of a vallecular cyst: a case report. Ear Nose Throat J 2005;84(3):170–2.
4. Hockstein NG, Nolan JP, O'Malley BW Jr, et al. Robotic microlaryngeal surgery: a technical feasibility study using the daVinci surgical robot and an airway mannequin. Laryngoscope 2005;115(5):780–5.
5. Boehm DH, Arnold MB, Detter C, et al. Incorporating robotics into an open-heart program. Surg Clin North Am 2003;83(6):1369–80.
6. Binder J, Brautigam R, Jonas D, et al. Robotic surgery in urology: fact or fantasy? BJU Int 2004;94(8):1183–7.
7. Advincula AP, Falcone T. Laparoscopic robotic gynecologic surgery. Obstet Gynecol Clin North Am 2004;31(3):599–609, ix–x.
8. Jacobsen G, Berger R, Horgan S. The role of robotic surgery in morbid obesity. J Laparoendosc Adv Surg Tech A 2003;13(4):279–83.
9. Hockstein NG, Nolan JP, O'Malley BW Jr, et al. Robot-assisted pharyngeal and laryngeal microsurgery: results of robotic cadaver dissections. Laryngoscope 2005;115(6):1003–8.
10. Hockstein NG, O'Malley BW Jr, Weinstein GS. Assessment of intraoperative safety in transoral robotic surgery. Laryngoscope 2006;116(2):165–8.
11. Weinstein GS, O'Malley BW Jr, Hockstein NG. Transoral robotic surgery: supraglottic laryngectomy in a canine model. Laryngoscope 2005;115(7):1315–9.
12. Hockstein NG, Weinstein GS, O'Malley BW Jr. Maintenance of hemostasis in transoral robotic surgery. ORL J Otorhinolaryngol Relat Spec 2005;67(4): 220–4.
13. O'Malley BW Jr, Weinstein GS, Snyder W, et al. Transoral robotic surgery (TORS) for base of tongue neoplasms. Laryngoscope 2006;116(8):1465–72.
14. Genden EM, Desai S, Sung CK. Transoral robotic surgery for the management of head and neck cancer: a preliminary experience. Head Neck 2009;31(3): 283–9.
15. Weinstein GS, O'Malley BW Jr, Snyder W, et al. Transoral robotic surgery: radical tonsillectomy. Arch Otolaryngol Head Neck Surg 2007;133(12):1220–6.
16. Boudreaux BA, Rosenthal EL, Magnuson JS, et al. Robot-assisted surgery for upper aerodigestive tract neoplasms. Arch Otolaryngol Head Neck Surg 2009; 135(4):397–401.
17. Holsinger FC, Sweeney AD, Jantharapattana K, et al. The emergence of endoscopic head and neck surgery. Curr Oncol Rep 2010;12(3):216–22.

18. Kang SW, Jeong JJ, Yun JS, et al. Gasless endoscopic thyroidectomy using trans-axillary approach; surgical outcome of 581 patients. Endocr J 2009;56(3): 361–9.
19. Holsinger FC, Terris DJ, Kuppersmith RB. Robotic thyroidectomy: operative technique using a transaxillary endoscopic approach without CO2 insufflation. Otolaryngol Clin North Am 2010;43(2):381–8, ix–x.
20. Klapan I, Vranjes Z, Risavi R, et al. Computer-assisted surgery and computer-assisted telesurgery in otorhinolaryngology. Ear Nose Throat J 2006;85(5): 318–21.
21. Breitenstein S, Nocito A, Puhan M, et al. Robotic-assisted versus laparoscopic cholecystectomy: outcome and cost analyses of a case-matched control study. Ann Surg 2008;247(6):987–93.
22. Bolenz C, Gupta A, Hotze T, et al. Cost comparison of robotic, laparoscopic, and open radical prostatectomy for prostate cancer. Eur Urol 2010;57(3):453–8.
23. Patel HR, Linares A, Joseph JV. Robotic and laparoscopic surgery: cost and training. Surg Oncol 2009;18(3):242–6.
24. Vicini C, Dallan I, Canzi P, et al. Transoral robotic tongue base resection in obstructive sleep apnoea-hypopnoea syndrome: a preliminary report. ORL J Otorhinolaryngol Relat Spec 2010;72(1):22–7.
25. O'Malley BW Jr, Weinstein GS. Robotic skull base surgery: preclinical investigations to human clinical application. Arch Otolaryngol Head Neck Surg 2007; 133(12):1215–9.
26. O'Malley BW Jr, Weinstein GS. Robotic anterior and midline skull base surgery: preclinical investigations. Int J Radiat Oncol Biol Phys 2007;69(Suppl 2): S125–128.
27. Hanna EY, Holsinger C, DeMonte F, et al. Robotic endoscopic surgery of the skull base: a novel surgical approach. Arch Otolaryngol Head Neck Surg 2007; 133(12):1209–14.
28. Lee JY, O'Malley BW, Newman JG, et al. Transoral robotic surgery of craniocervical junction and atlantoaxial spine: a cadaveric study. J Neurosurg Spine 2010;12(1):13–8.

Training and Simulation in Otolaryngology

Gregory J. Wiet, MD[a,b,*], Don Stredney, MA[a,b,c], Dinah Wan, MD[d]

KEYWORDS

- Simulation technology • Training simulation • Education
- Surgical simulation • Medical simulation • ENT simulation
- Continuing education

THE NEED FOR SURGICAL SIMULATION IN OTOLARYNGOLOGY

Despite ever improving less-invasive medical treatment regimens, surgical intervention is still required for many health conditions. As an example, disorders of the temporal bone affect millions of patients in the United States[1] and many require surgical intervention for resolution. To gain surgical proficiency, trainees must possess comprehension of the complex anatomy and associated pathology of the temporal bone. This knowledge must be integrated with refined microsurgical technical skill. This proficiency requires many hours of deliberate practice and considerable clinical experience. Surgical training requires at least 5 years under current methods at a cost of approximately $80,000 per year per resident.[2] Conventional temporal bone laboratories with related equipment cost more than a $1 million to construct and are expensive to maintain (D.B. Welling, personal communication, 2010; recently outfitted complete temporal bone laboratory with 12 stations with instructor station, ~$2 million). Several factors contribute to inefficiencies in traditional training methodologies, adversely impacting the overall cost of health care. The barriers to progress include less time available for teaching and learning, limitations of instructional resources, and perhaps most importantly the lack of a uniform objective assessment of technical skills.

Less Time Available for Teaching and Learning

There are a few limiting factors adversely influencing the amount of time available for teaching in training centers. First, as health care costs continue to escalate, financial

[a] Department of Otolaryngology, The Ohio State University, College of Medicine, 915 Olentangy River Road, Suite 4000, Columbus, OH 43212, USA
[b] Department of Biomedical Informatics, The Ohio State University, 3190 Graves Hall, 333 West Tenth Avenue, Columbus, OH 43210, USA
[c] Ohio Supercomputer Center, The Ohio State University, 1224 Kinnear Road, Columbus, OH 43212, USA
[d] The Ohio State University College of Medicine, 370 West 9th Avenue, Columbus, OH 43210, USA
* Corresponding author. Department of Otolaryngology, The Ohio State University, and Nationwide Children's Hospital, 700 Children's Drive, Columbus, OH 43205.
E-mail address: Gregory.Wiet@nationwidechildrens.org

Otolaryngol Clin N Am 44 (2011) 1333–1350
doi:10.1016/j.otc.2011.08.009
0030-6665/11/$ – see front matter © 2011 Elsevier Inc. All rights reserved.

pressures come to bear on teaching physicians. An increased demand for "clinical effi-ciency" in the operating room and outpatient clinics limits the amount of time faculty can devote to actually teaching. Second, the restrictions of duty hours for trainees imposed to reduce fatigue and related errors also limit the amount of time available for hands-on learning. This presents a disassociation of the traditional model of "apprentice and master" introduced by Halsted and Osler in the late 1800s. Third, this reduction leads to the concern for insufficient development of technical skills acquired in the operating room and requires learning and practice outside of patient care.

Limitations of Instructional Resources

A few limitations of instructional resources are apparent. First, there is a reduced avail-ability of cadaveric material, the previous gold standard for practicing technical maneuvers outside of patient care. Ethical procurement and proper disposal present necessary and continuous challenges. Sources of human material are no longer avail-able from foreign countries and fewer patients and their families are consenting to donation. Second, there is reduced access to faculty expertise, a key instructional resource. Because of financial pressures, faculty have fewer hours available for teaching, especially for critical assessment during formative development that requires considerable time. With financial pressure for more clinical productivity to maintain previous income levels, the numbers of teaching faculty are decreasing. Finally, of continuing concern is exposure to hazardous materials including pathogens present in cadaveric specimens (eg, hepatitis B and C, prion-derived illness,[3] and HIV infection) and increased exposure to formalin[4,5] that present increased dangers to health. Use of simulation technologies presents the capacity to greatly mitigate these limitations of instructional resources.

Lack of a Uniform Objective Assessment of Technical Skills

Perhaps most importantly, there is a lack of uniform and objective standardized metrics for use in the assessment of technical skills. Without standardized metrics, uniform formative feedback during training and measurement of professional technical proficiency is not being achieved. This has resulted because no methodology previ-ously existed to objectively apply metrics that were valid, reliable, and practical.

Recently, it has been asserted that today's training methodologies are antiquated and that a new balance between patient safety and physician training is necessary.[6] A more standardized and structured approach to curriculum development, continuous assessment of skills, constructive feedback, and provision for deliberate practice outside of direct patient care are necessary. Elements required in technical skills development include not only facility to practice psychomotor skills but also elements that reinforce adequate knowledge of a specific procedure, such as relevant anatomy, instrumentation, indications, complications, and postoperative management. This reinforcement requires demonstration of a procedure, delineation of the key steps, assurance of comprehension of the key steps, and single component mastery fol-lowed by entire procedure mastery. Formative continuous and summative assess-ment of skill is necessary. Simulation technologies provide the mechanism by which this reinforcement can be achieved with efficient use of the expert.

SIMULATION IN SUPPORT OF TECHNICAL SKILLS TRAINING

Simulation environments are uniquely suited to allow deliberate practice in a non-threatening environment (**Fig. 1**). For these systems to be effective they require the

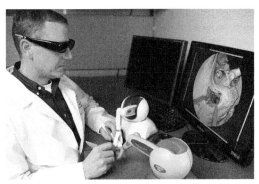

Fig. 1. User in current temporal bone simulator from The Ohio State University. Interface includes stereo visual and dual haptic feedback devices for procedural interaction.

integration of automated expert feedback based on rigorous standards and more than just an environment for the replication of a real-world task.

Johnson[7] points out that simulation is particularly suited to provide (1) errors without putting patients at risk (ie, error-based learning); (2) objective performance measurements and a standardized learning process; and (3) that a realistic simulation provides "situational context," with more effective reification of the elements to be learned.

This article presents the issues of applying advanced computing and simulation environments for supporting technical skills training and meeting the proscribed criteria established by Johnson. It should be noted that this discussion excludes other avenues used for simulation training, including mannequins and box-trainers. The main focus of this article is simulation environments that support the development of technical skills needed to successfully execute surgical procedures and that integrate automated standards.

TECHNICAL SKILLS ASSESSMENT AND SIMULATION

The need for accurate assessment of skill is paramount for any effective training and maintenance of skill. Two types of assessment are defined and necessary: formative assessment for improvement and development and summative assessment for evaluation of competency. Formative assessments need to be specific and concrete to suggest actions for improvement (feedback).[8] Summative assessment is data driven and requires statistical rigor and validation to make a valid judgment of an individual's skill level. The goal with respect to simulation is to demonstrate that competency within the simulator translates into competency in the clinical realm. Competency can be assessed in the simulator by objective measures, such as time to task, error rate, and economy of movement. For this level of assessment to occur, establishment of standards of competency must be developed. Minimally acceptable performance needs to be determined by a panel of experts. These benchmarks must then be established within the simulation and validated in that context by the experts. The inclusion of expert-defined benchmarks helps provide a theoretical link to patient outcomes in the early adaption and adoption of a technical skills training simulator.

Well-designed simulators are posed to provide a paradigm shift in objective assessment of technical skill. Current methods to assess technical competency are seriously flawed and continue to receive little attention from certification bodies.[9] The core competencies defined by the Accreditation Council for Graduate Medical Education do not provide an adequate, objective assessment of technical skill. The reasons for this are many. However, the largest roadblock to improving technical skills assessment is the lack of an objective methodology that is reliable, valid, and practical. Reliability refers to consistency, repeatability, and dependability of the measures. Validity refers to the concept of a metric actually measuring what it is supposed to measure and able to be defined by criterion (correlates with other measures), construct (correlates with level of training), content (reflects content of domain), and face (extent of measure reflecting real life situation). Use of simulators in domains other than otolaryngology has been shown to provide valid, reliable, and practical assessment of technical skill.[9] It is imperative that the field of otolaryngology follows suit in this area of objective assessment.

Technical skills assessment requires a gold standard with which other assessment methodologies can be compared. No truly objective, validated assessments are widely available in otolaryngology. Validated assessment tools are beginning to emerge through the use of expert opinions and surveys.[10–12] The otologic experience lags behind that which has been established in sinus surgery (see the discussion of the Endoscopic Sinus Surgery Simulator [ES3]). In the context of otologic surgery, these assessment tools are still cumbersome, ill defined, and impractical to administer; they often require long hours of expert review of individual performances and validation. As a result study sizes are small. With respect to that developed for the sinus surgery simulator studies, most are small and further limited because of the cost of the simulator hardware. Only through large-scale, multiinstitutional studies can these tools be more standardized, rigorously studied, validated, and accepted.

The establishment of technical skills assessment tools with expert defined metrics integrated into a simulation-based training system will be the underpinning for proficiency-based training programs. Brydges and coworkers[13] describe a methodology for developing such a simulation-based training program where trainees progress from less to more technically demanding skills and tasks, only after achieving defined criteria. This methodology is, in a sense, implicit in the "apprentice and master" training system but not well defined. The current execution has been marked by nonstandardized and subjective influences with the ultimate criteria being the completion of a prescribed time in training or "adequate number of procedures." This current concept of surgical skills training and assessment does not provide objective and valid measures of performance. Simulation-based training and assessment provides the means by which valid and objective measures can be instituted and provides a safe environment for surgical trainees to assess their performance rigorously without risk to patients.[14] The experience with the ES3, although on a small scale, has demonstrated that this can be accomplished within the otolaryngology community.

SIMULATION SYSTEMS IN OTOLARYNGOLOGY

Since the introduction of simulation in medicine, otolaryngology has increasingly been involved in promoting its development and validation, most notably in endoscopic sinus surgery and temporal bone surgery. A complete review of these two areas was recently published.[15,16] The following provides a brief summary of past developments and more current progress.

ENDOSCOPIC SINUS SURGERY SIMULATOR

The ES3 was the first sinus surgery simulator developed and remains a leading system with several validation studies completed.[17] Inspired by aviation training simulators for military aircraft, the ES3 was developed between 1995 and 1998 by Lockheed Martin, in association with the University of Washington, The Ohio State University (OSU), and the Ohio Supercomputer Center, with sponsorship from the US Army Medical Research and Materiel Command.[18] The ES3 was first used in the Army in 1997 and gained popularity among medical students and residents within the armed forces. The simulation system involves CT-derived three-dimensional paranasal sinus anatomy models and interactions with a virtual endoscopic instrument with haptic feedback. The ES3 uses an "expert surgical assistant" that interprets multimodal input to provide automated feedback to the user and warnings as critical structures are approached. It also allows the user to query the system regarding relevant anatomy and procedural maneuvers.[19] Yale University has developed a state-of-the-art curriculum to standardize training on the ES3 regardless of level, available on a compact disk. The ES3 consortium is currently led by Albert Einstein College of Medicine and includes the Agency for Healthcare Research and Quality (funding); Yale University (curriculum development); New York University Medical Center; New York Eye and Ear Infirmary; Mount Sinai Medical Center (data collection); and the University of Washington–Human Interface Technology Laboratory (web database) (**Fig. 2**).

"The ES3 is one of the few virtual reality simulators with a comprehensive validation record,"[15,16] a notion that allows it to be claimed as one of the leading ESS simulation systems. An initial study demonstrating construct validity of the ES3 showed significant correlation between performance on the ES3 and performance on other validated tests of innate ability in psychomotor, visuospatial, and perceptual capacities (to parallel the ESS-required skill of two-handed coordination of surgical instruments in a three-dimensional space).[20] A second study compared the performance of medical students, otolaryngology residents, and attendings on the ES3. The ES3 was clearly able to distinguish between the three levels in initial trials, with the expert performing at the highest level, followed by residents, then medical students. This study also showed that all groups achieved a remarkably similar plateau score by the tenth trial on the simulator, demonstrating the ability of the ES3 to consistently achieve a standard performance goal in users.[21] The most recent validation study (Virtual Reality to Operating Room), which provides the strongest clinical correlation, evaluates whether training on the ES3 translates to improved performance in actual surgery. This study showed that otolaryngology junior residents who received both conventional sinus surgery training and ES3 training (experimental group) performed significantly better than residents who received only conventional training (control group). Improved

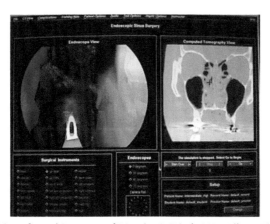

Fig. 2. ES3 visual interface. (*Courtesy of* Marvin P. Fried, MD, Albert Einstein College of Medicine.)

performance in the experimental group includes significantly shorter operating time, demonstration of higher confidence, better skills in instrument manipulation, and fewer technical errors.[15,16] Of interest, the ES3 has also been shown to be an effective tool in training ophthalmology residents in endoscopic endonasal dacryocystorhinostomy at the Albert Einstein College of Medicine, effectively extending its use beyond the field of otolaryngology.[22] The limitations of the ES3 are that it is no longer in production and there are only a handful of systems in existence. Additionally, there has been no update to the underlying technology supporting the system since its inception over a decade ago. Dr Marvin Fried of Albert Einstein College of Medicine has continued to champion the use of this simulator and has been a pioneer in its application (**Fig. 3**).

OTHER ESS SIMULATORS

Although the ES3 remains the primary ESS simulation system in the United States, several other ESS simulators are worthy of mention. The University of Hamburg-Eppendorf group in Germany (developers of the VOXEL-MAN TempoSurg simulator) recently developed a new paranasal sinus surgery simulator that is compatible with standard personal computer hardware. This system uses three-dimensional models of human skulls obtained from high-resolution CT images with mucosa and vital relevant organs added manually. It uses a lower-cost haptic feedback device to promote affordability. Learning effects of this simulation have yet to be quantified.[23] The Innovation Center for Computer Assisted Surgery group (ICCAS) at the Medical Faculty of the University of Leipzig, Germany, is also developing a virtual reality functional ES3 and a transphenoidal pituitary surgery simulator. The ICCAS projects generally place a stronger emphasis on clinical applications (ie, preoperative planning and intraoperative guidance) rather than training. Another group at Colombia is using "telesimulation" to create a virtual reality tool aiding trainees in resource-limited countries to gain skills to perform functional endoscopic sinus surgery. Their project, the Web Environment for Surgery Skills Training on Otolaryngology, uses an Internet-based educational cycle that simulates the stages of a real procedure. This system still requires work in its development, but represents a valuable concept of telesimulation to promote distance learning in disadvantaged countries.[24] Researchers at Stanford have recently implemented a sinus surgery simulation environment that introduces automatically derived data sets from preoperative, patient-specific imaging.[25]

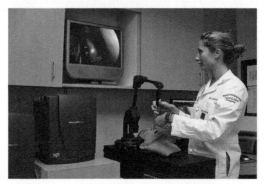

Fig. 3. User in ES3 simulator. (*Courtesy of* Marvin P. Fried, MD, Albert Einstein College of Medicine.)

SIMULATION OF TEMPORAL BONE SURGERY
Traditional Media in the Otologic Curriculum

To date, temporal bone surgery has been learned through contemporary media: textbooks and atlases,[26–29] illustrations, CD-ROMS,[30,31] models,[32,33] and cadaver dissections.[34,35] Although CD-ROMs provided a cost-effective solution through the integration of photographs, illustrations, movies, computer graphics, and tomographic images, the solutions from interaction remain predetermined and provide limited, if any, task fidelity (ie, correlation between the training and performance environment). Selections are from a limited number of choices, are schematic in representation, and the results are not unique to the individual.

It is difficult to achieve a consummate comprehension of the subtle spatial relationships required for temporal bone surgery without diligent studies through dissection over a period of 4 to 5 years.[34,35] To facilitate understanding of the intricacies of the regional anatomy of the temporal bone, some authors have presented techniques for tissue preservation and display.[32] The resulting displays provide the student with only limited and passive means to study the intricate relationships of structures found in the temporal bone. In addition, the physical limitation of the material, associated risk of infection (HIV, hepatitis B and C), exposure to formalin, and decreasing availability make this method increasingly problematic. To increase the availability of material and reduce the risks of infection, Pettigrew[33] introduced a plastic model of the otic capsule and middle ear for drilling practice. These models are structurally realistic and serve as substitute materials for drilling practice. However, plastic models are subject to similar physical limitations as cadaver specimens (ie, to start over, a new plastic specimen must be used), and provide a limited force correlate (ie, biofidelity) to actual bone because of the homogeneity of the plastics.

Use of Computer Simulations in Histopathologic and Morphologic Studies

Three-dimensional reconstructions from CT have been extensively integrated with computer-aided design techniques to provide a non–real-time system for use in the diagnosis and surgical planning of craniofacial disorders.[36] Methods for characterizing the morphology and histopathology of the temporal bone soon followed.[35] Subsequently, these methods were combined with computer-aided reconstruction techniques for visualization and morphometric analysis.[37–48] Although specimen preparation and integration of the photomicrographs through manual methods was time intensive, the advantage of three-dimensional reconstructions to demonstrate subtle morphologic relationships and changes clearly became evident. More recently, several groups have used photomicrographs to create elegant data sets of the human temporal bone.[49] Although providing exquisite detail and near natural coloration, these preparations take considerable time and effort, and consequently provide limited variance.

Harada and coworkers[50] first introduced the concept of exploiting three-dimensional volumetric reconstructions from CT for emulating drilling and exposing the intricate regional anatomy of the temporal bone. However, because of the computational overhead of volumetric representation at the time, real-time interactions were unavailable. Subsequently, surface-based (isosurfaces) approaches were predominantly used for modeling structure to exploit the hardware-accelerated surface rendering techniques that have been developed for other applications, such as video gaming. Similar techniques using reconstructions from histologic sections to derive isosurfaces have focused on clarifying the spatial relationships of the regional anatomy.[46,51–53] Stereo presentations of surface-based models acquired from the Visible Human Project[54,55] have been presented for transpetrosal, retrosigmoid, and middle fossa approaches to the cerebropontine angle.[56] Although surface-based representations of soft tissues and bone structures have been developed, the systems do not provide haptic feedback to the user, and only provide a schematic emulation of dissection and surgical technique. The development of stereo volumetric, physically based simulations has been presented.[57–59] These systems do not support real-time viewing and aural simulation. Although volumetric data sets have been integrated, no multiscale data (ie, data acquired at multiple scales) has been reported. Agus[58] has extensively explored efforts to present secondary characteristics, such as bleeding, debris formation, and fluid flow simulation. Ray-casting techniques have been developed to provide stereo simulations of cutting and drilling based on reconstructions from CT.[60] Although all investigators present initial enthusiasm from local surgeons and residents, local or extensive multi-institutional studies have not been conducted to validate the efficacy of these systems compared with traditional methods of training and assessment.

CURRENT SYSTEMS
Stanford University

The temporal bone simulation system developed at Stanford University uses CT data with hybrid volume and surface-based three-dimensional rendering, and a haptic interface providing force feedback and vibration. The haptic interface is networked, allowing a trainee to "feel" forces and maneuvers being applied by an expert in a linked system.[61] The simulator has demonstrated construct validity with a study showing significantly different global scores received by experienced users compared with novice users performing a mastoidectomy on the simulator.[62] A validation study demonstrating translation of the simulator's beneficial learning effects to improved performance in the operating room is still in process. Stanford's group places special emphasis on promoting independent learning on the simulator, eliminating the need for constant supervision by an instructor. Sewell and coworkers[63] presented specific metrics integrated into the simulator. Implementation of these metrics allowed the simulator to provide instant automated instructional feedback to the user. Integrated metrics include drilling and suctioning techniques, bone removal, facial nerve exposure, and drill forces and velocities.

The Ohio State University

The temporal bone simulator developed at OSU Medical Center in conjunction with the Ohio Supercomputer Center also uses a hybrid renderer similar to that used in the Stanford system (see **Fig. 1**; **Figs. 4–6**). The OSU system is being developed under funding from the National Institutes of Health and National Institute on Deafness and Other Communication Disorders. The difference in approaches between the two systems centers on how the bone is rendered. The OSU simulator used direct volume rendering, whereas the Stanford simulator uses a surface-based approach. The OSU simulator uses three interfaces to create a seamless environment, including a visual component emulating a stereomicroscope, a haptic component with force feedback emulating drilling burrs and irrigation and suction devices, and an aural element producing drill and suction sounds that spatially correlate with drill pressure and speed.[64] It also integrates an "intelligent tutor" that highlights relevant anatomic structures within the temporal bone on the user's prompt. To provide an exceptional contextual realism[7] the OSU system places special emphasis on structural and contextual realism. Recent additions include enhancement of fluid rendering (bleeding effects, meniscus rendering, and refraction) and a shading model to enhance wet surfaces.[65,66] Preliminary trials show that this simulator has reached the standard of

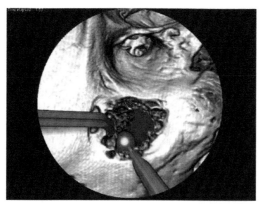

Fig. 4. View from OSU temporal bone simulator demonstrating interactive fluidic effects of suction and irrigation and bleeding.

development to be used in otology residency training curriculums.[67–69] Furthermore, the system is currently completing a large multiinstitutional (10 sites and 70 study subjects) trial evaluating performance outcomes of medical students and residents. This study looked at training in the simulator versus cadaveric temporal bone specimens (**Fig. 7**). Current efforts seek to address identified limitations, which include a seamless hierarchical representation of data acquired at multiple resolutions, a distance field approach for rendering key structures in an intelligent tutor,[70,71] and automated assessments derived from expert validated metrics.[12]

VOXEL-MAN, University of Hamburg-Eppendorf, Germany

The VOXEL-MAN TempoSurg simulator (Spiggle and Theis, Overath, Germany; www. uke.de/voxel-man) is currently the only commercial temporal bone simulator on the

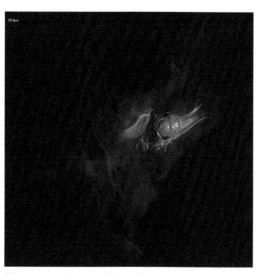

Fig. 5. Image of cochlea using distance field effect to delineate and emphasize associated structures and cavities.

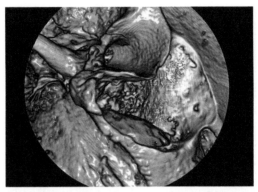

Fig. 6. View from OSU temporal bone simulator showing thinning near tegmen and coloration of underlying sigmoid sinus.

market. Similar to existing temporal bone simulators, VOXEL-MAN uses three-dimensional temporal bone models derived from high-resolution CT and a haptic device providing force feedback. Images are displayed stereoscopically through a mirror. The most recent validation study involved 20 otolaryngology physicians of varying seniority who completed a self-evaluation of skill level and subsequently performed a mastoidectomy on the simulator.[72] Two expert raters blindly assessed video recordings of their performance and gave an overall impression score and a score for specific domains (ie, flow of operation and respect for tissues) for added objectivity. Results demonstrated significant positive correlation between participants' self-ratings of skill level and scores given by the expert raters. There was also significant positive correlation between the overall impression scores and the total score obtained from the specific domains. An earlier validation study involving otolaryngology surgeons at the University of Toronto yielded more ambiguous findings.[73] In that study, videos were recorded of novice and experienced surgeons performing dissection on the simulator or on a cadaveric temporal bone. Expert raters were able to discriminate novice from experienced trainees at a significant level only on cadaveric bones. There was also a trend toward discrimination in the simulator recordings, although this correlation was not significant. The use of expert raters to review performance in these studies was time consuming and lent itself to subjective biases.

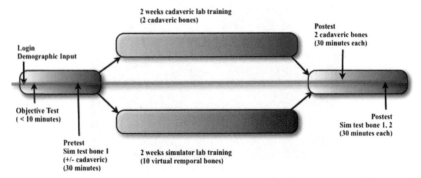

Fig. 7. Diagram of protocol used in multiinstitutional study of OSU temporal bone project.

Integrated Environment for the Rehearsal and Planning of Surgical Intervention Project, European Union

The Integrated Environment for the Rehearsal and Planning of Surgical Intervention Project is led by a consortium of European physicians and technologists and is funded by the European Commission. This group produced a temporal bone simulator that uses stereoscopically rendered three-dimensional models of temporal bones derived from CT and a haptic feedback device. The three main uses of their system include (1) preoperation planning using patient-specific data, (2) surgical simulation, and (3) education and training.[59,74] The simulator functionalities were divided into fast and slow subsystems, each responsible for different tasks. Agus and coworkers[57] used this dichotomy to decouple the simulation on a multiprocessor personal computer platform. In another report detailing the performance of a canal wall-up mastoidectomy on the simulator, it showed strong three-dimensional simulation and dust and color representation during the first part of the procedure, but poor simulation when approaching the deeper portions of the model because of lack of haptic feedback from soft tissue and underrepresentation of anatomy in the pneumatized bone.[75]

Other Temporal Bone Surgery Simulators

The ICCAS at the University of Leipzig has developed a patient-specific high-resolution ear model, the main purpose of which is surgical guidance. They use a high-resolution microMR model overlaid onto the patient CT image, transforming the patient image into a high-resolution model in a course-to-fine approach. The group is also working on a model-guided mastoid surgery, which uses a high-resolution patient-specific CT image of the mastoid region to conduct preoperative planning. This program offers such applications as "navigated control," where the drill is automatically switched off when approaching risky structures. Again, most of the work from ICCAS focuses on clinical applications, such as surgical workflow, which uses simulation to quantify and automate surgical strategies.

Finally, Sorensen and coworkers[76] have compiled an exquisite high-resolution data set derived from a single cadaveric specimen. This data set provides an unprecedented image resolution. It has been subsequently integrated into a temporal bone simulator (**Fig. 8**) and is available for free download at http://www.alexandra.dk/ves/index.htm.

Simulation in Other Areas of Otolaryngology

The University of Western Ontario recently developed a three-dimensional virtual reality myringotomy simulator using haptic feedback. This system is one of the first

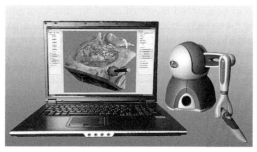

Fig. 8. Visible Ear Simulator. (*Courtesy of* Mads Sorensen, MD, Rigshospitalet, Copenhagen, Denmark.)

virtual reality simulators in outer and middle ear surgery and demonstrated good-to-excellent face validity with high consistency in initial validation trials.[77]

A group at the University of Bern in Switzerland has created a simulator that provides surgical planning for anterior and lateral skull-based surgery. CT, magnetic resonance imaging, and angiography-derived images of the skull base are overlaid onto the surgical view using the simulator. This system provides a navigation system that is shown to improve surgical outcomes including decreased surgery time and less invasive approaches.[78]

Efforts have also been made toward developing the computer-aided design–computer-aided manufacturing technique in mandibular reconstruction surgery. In this approach, the patient's CT image is transferred into a software application that allows the design of patient-specific plates or titanium membranes for optimal reconstruction. This approach has been shown to improve operative time and accuracy of surgical technique.[79,80]

DISCUSSION

Clearly, emulation of the complex interaction of human surgery is daunting. However disparate many of these developments have been, all have presented improvements to various elements. These improvements provide strong evidence of emerging end-to-end comprehensive systems. The following presents a discussion regarding continued and emerging influences and trends for further integration of simulation in the resident curriculum.

Advantages of Emerging Technology

Emerging technologies, most notably in graphical processing units, provide unprecedented opportunities for advancements in simulation environments. Reduced costs in graphical processing units and multicore technologies serve to promote the dissemination and adoption of simulation technologies. Whereas initial simulations in the mid-1990s required hardware environments in the hundreds of thousands of dollars, more complete and complex systems are generally available today for tens of thousands of dollars. This drop in the cost, by an order of magnitude, allows for increased participation by a broader and more diverse community of users, and subsequently can serve to promote the adaptation of simulation use.

The increased processor speed and capacity allow for more complex data sets to be loaded into memory. Advances in imaging technologies and integration of data will continue. As imaging technologies become more sophisticated, there will be an increase in the precision that data is acquired, in the types of data acquired at multiple scales, and in the integration of data from different modalities. These emerging techniques will lead to unprecedented levels of detail in structural representation of the regional anatomy. As these techniques are translated to safe, nonirradiating methods, there will be an increase in the use of simulation environments for precise preoperative assessment and planning.[81]

Increases in processing capacity will continue to exert positive influences on representation. These advances in processing size and power will lead to unprecedented levels of realism and dynamic interaction. Increased processor capabilities and speed provide new avenues to achieve increasingly realistic representations, providing more realistic lighting and coloration models and methods to modify representations to guide the user's focal attention (see **Figs. 4–6**).[70] These effects can be amortized by using the same data sets, allowing for depiction of various levels of detail, from schematic through realistic.[65,70] This capability allows for the amortization of acquisition costs by expanding the use of the single data set to include introductory training sessions, intermediate training sessions, and more complex procedural training at high levels of realism.

In addition, subtle interaction, such as tissue deformation[82–84] and fluidics,[65] previously unavailable is beginning to become achievable (see **Fig. 4**). These improvements in contextual realism open opportunities for more advanced training and interests in preoperative assessment, including the presentation of representations of adverse consequences. These realistic contextual representations can directly affect the motivation for users. Further studies will help to pursue correlation between the simulation (training) environments, including depiction of various outcomes measured in the performance.

Interfaces

Haptic interfaces need to be further developed, or new methods to provide dexterous interaction need to become available. For instance, cutting (scissoring) and pinching (fine grasping) need to be developed. This would allow for an expanded repertoire of surgical techniques and interaction, and may lead to new interfaces for robotic intervention.[81] As these simulation interfaces improve, they will become more widely used to study surgical innovation and the pursuit of new operative techniques. Coupled with advances in emulating soft tissue deformation, these systems will provide unprecedented levels of realism to reach the objective of presenting a strong situational context.

User Monitoring

With the establishment of objective standards, the authors foresee improved assessment of proficiency. This includes the deliberate translation of expert assessment into objective automated assessments of proficiency and the use of more objective assessment in a more continuous fashion.

Furthermore, they anticipate increased use of physiologic metrics of users. The metrics will be used to establish levels of attention, motivation, and perseveration during various conditions of difficulty. As simulation increasingly supports multiple cases to present a wider variance to the user, systems that integrate and capture physiologic metrics will provide sophisticated vehicles to better characterize shared levels of difficulty, and how the user responds to adverse events encountered in a simulation.

Factors Limiting Progress

In the authors' experience, the most limiting factor adversely effecting progress is the lack of objective standards. Standardized metrics form the basis for an objective tool to evaluate different training modalities and support standardized curriculum development. Both functions are essential not only for proper development of proficiency, but also to more effectively evaluate simulation environments. Furthermore, establishing quantitative objective standards is crucial to promoting a community that uses standardize metrics for proficiency assessment.

A second factor impeding progress is reluctance to participate in formative development studies. It takes considerable time and effort for the iterative development and validation of systems required to emulate the complex environment and interactions of surgery. However, many possible participants expect systems to be further developed and validated, and are unwilling to volunteer time and effort for early development. Yet, for development and validation to properly occur, multicenter consortiums and government funding sources must be willing to invest the time and effort and support in formative development to help realize the full potential of emerging systems. Potential study subjects, trainees, and experts need time and support for these endeavors. In the authors' experience, many individuals have limited time to participate in developmental research.[85] Those who do participate are volunteers with limited, if any, compensation. Furthermore, institutional review boards stipulate anonymity. In addition, the institutional review board protocol must ensure the prevention of coercion of residents in participation, effort, or study completion. All of these issues can adversely influence motivation of study subjects and significantly impact study outcomes.

SUMMARY

Simulation technology provides the platform for which efficient and objective evaluation of technical skills can be implemented. The development of such systems for uniform, metrics-based training and assessment is crucial for surgical training to progress to a new level of competence and accountability. Pressures from both society at large and from within the healthcare community have reached a critical mass that is now forcing change on the training and assessment aspects of surgery. The onus is on the otolaryngology community to become involved in the development of simulation systems for standardized, metric-driven training and technical skills assessment. It is not only in the development of these systems that the responsibility lays, but also in the scientifically rigorous evaluation and iterative refinement. The use of simulation technology truly has the potential for paradigm shift from methodologies for training and assessment developed in the 1800s to move forward in a practical and efficient manner.

ACKNOWLEDGMENTS

Portions of this research, Validation/Dissemination of Virtual Temporal Bone Dissection, is supported by a grant from the National Institute on Deafness and Other Communication Disorders, of the National Institutes of Health, 1 R01 DC06458-01A1. The authors thank Thomas Kerwin, BS, for help with preparation of the manuscript.

REFERENCES

1. National Institute on Deafness and Other Communication Disorders. 2010. Available at: http://www.nidcd.nih.gov/health/statistics/hearing.asp. Accessed May 27, 2011.
2. Williams TE, Santiani B, Thomas A, et al. The impending shortage and the estimated cost of training the future surgical workforce. Ann Surg 2009;27:590–7.
3. Scott A, De R, Sadek SA, et al. Temporal bone dissection: a possible route for prion transmission? J Laryngol Otol 2001;115(5):374–5.
4. NIOSH. 2010. Available at: http://www.cdc.gov/niosh/npg/npgd0294.html. Accessed May 27, 2011.
5. Pettigrew AM. 2010. Available at: www.temporal-bone.com/plastic.htm. Accessed May 27, 2011.
6. Grantcharov TP, Reznick RK. Teaching procedural skills. BMJ 2008;336:1129–31.
7. Johnson E. Surgical simulators and simulated surgeons: reconstituting medical practice and practitioners in simulations. Soc Stud Sci 2007;37(4):585–608.
8. Michelson JD, Manning L. Competency assessment in simulation-based procedural education. Am J Surg 2008;196:609–15.
9. Sidhu RS, Grober ED, Musselman LJ, et al. Assessing competency in surgery: Where to begin? Surgery 2004;135(1):6–20.

10. Butler NN, Wiet GJ. Reliability of the Welling Scale (WS1) for rating temporal bone dissection performance. Laryngoscope 2007;117(10):1803–8.
11. Laeeq K, Bhatti NI, Carey JP, et al. Pilot testing of an assessment tool for competency in mastoidectomy. Laryngoscope 2009;119:2402–10.
12. Wan D, Wiet GJ, Welling B, et al. Creating a cross-institutional grading scale for temporal bone dissection. Laryngoscope 2010;120(7):1422–7.
13. Brydges R, Kurahashi A, Brummer V, et al. Developing criteria for proficiency-based training of surgical technical skills using simulation: changes in performances as a function of training year. J Am Coll Surg 2008;206:205–11.
14. Tavakol M, Mohagheghi MA, Dennick R. Assessing the skills of surgical residents using simulation. J Surg Educ 2008;65(2):77–83.
15. Fried MP, Sadoughi B, Gibber MJ, et al. From virtual reality to the operating room: the endoscopic sinus surgery simulator experiment. Otolaryngol Head Neck Surg 2010;142:202–7.
16. Fried MP, Wiet GJ, Sadoughi B. Simulation and haptics in otolaryngology training. In: Flint PW, Haughey BH, Lund VJ, et al, editors. Cummings otolaryngology – head and neck surgery. 5th edition. Philadelphia: Mosby; 2010. p. 45–51.
17. Gallagher AG. VR to OR. Presented at the Medicine Meets Virtual Reality 11 Newport Beach (CA), February 2003.
18. Edmond CV, Heskamp D, Sluis D, et al. ENT endoscopic surgical training simulator. Stud Health Technol Inform 1997;39:518–28.
19. Billinghurst M, Savage J, Oppenheimer P, et al. The expert surgical assistant. An intelligent virtual environment with multimodal input. Stud Health Technol Inform 1996;29:590–607.
20. Arora H, Uribe J, Ralph W, et al. Assessment of construct validity of the endoscopic sinus surgery simulator. Arch Otolaryngol Head Neck Surg 2005;131:217–21.
21. Fried MP, Sadoughi B, Weghorst SJ, et al. Construct validity of the endoscopic sinus surgery simulator: II. Assessment of discriminant validity and expert benchmarking. Arch Otolaryngol Head Neck Surg 2007;133(4):350–7.
22. Weiss M, Lauer SA, Fried MP, et al. Endoscopic endonasal surgery simulator as a training tool for ophthalmology residents. Ophthal Plast Reconstr Surg 2008;24(6):460–4.
23. Tolsdorff B, Pommert A, Hohne KH, et al. Virtual reality: a new paranasal sinus surgery simulator. Laryngoscope 2010;120:420–6.
24. Navarro AA, Hernandez CJ, Velez JA. Virtual surgical telesimulations in otolaryngology. Proc. Medicine Meets Virtual Reality 2005;13:353–5.
25. Wired Science. Virtual reality could keep you from being a surgical guinea pig. Wired.com Condé Nast Digital; 2009.
26. Donaldson JA. Surgical anatomy of the temporal bone. 4th edition. New York: Raven Press; 1992.
27. Glasscock ME, Shambaugh GE. Surgery of the ear. 4th edition. Philadelphia: WB Saunders; 1990.
28. Schuknecht HF, Gulya AJ. Anatomy of the temporal bone with surgical implications. Philadelphia: Lea & Febiger; 1986.
29. Swartz JD, Harnsberger HR. Imaging the temporal bone. 3rd edition. New York: Thieme; 1998.
30. Blevins NH, Jackler RK, Gralapp C. Temporal bone dissector: the interactive otology reference. CDROM. St. Louis: Mosby-Year Book; 1998.
31. Brodie H, Singh T. Temporal bone anatomy. CDROM. Sacramento (CA): University of California Davis Medical School; 1997.
32. Golding-Wood DG. Temporal bone dissection for display. J Laryngol Otol 1994;108(1):3–8.

33. Pettigrew. Available at:http://www.temporal-bone.com/plastic.htm. Accessed May 27, 2010.

34. Nelson RA. Temporal bone surgical dissection manual. 2nd edition. Los Angeles (CA): House Ear Institute; 1991.

35. Sando I, Takahara T, Doyle JD, et al. A method for the histopathological analysis of the temporal bone and the eustachian tube and its accessory structures. Ann Otol Rhinol Laryngol 1986;95:267–74.

36. Vannier MW, Marsh JL, Warren JO. Three-dimensional computer graphics for craniofacial surgical planning and evaluation. Comput Graph 1983;17(3):263–73.

37. Fujita S, Sando I. Postnatal development of the vestibular aqueduct in relation to the internal auditory canal, computer-aided three-dimensional reconstruction and measurement study. Ann Otol Rhinol Laryngol 1994;103:719–22.

38. Hinojosa R, Green D, Brecht K, et al. Otocephalus: histopathology and three-dimensional reconstruction. Otolaryngol Head Neck Surg 1996;114(1):44–53.

39. Ikui A, Sudo M, Sando I, et al. Postnatal change in angle between the tympanic annulus and surrounding structures-computer-aided three-dimensional reconstruction study. Ann Otol Rhinol Laryngol 1997;106:33–6.

40. Nakashima S, Sando I, Takahashi H, et al. Computer-aided 3-D reconstruction and measurement of the facial canal and facial nerve. Cross-sectional area and diameter: preliminary report. Laryngoscope 1993;103:1150–6.

41. Rosowski JJ, Dobrzenieki AB, Flandermeyer DT. Computer assisted three-dimensional reconstruction of normal and pathological human ears [abstract]. Otolaryngol Head Neck Surg 1996;115(2).

42. Rasmussion A, Modegaard J, Sorensen TS. Exploring parallel algorithms for volumetric mass-spring-damper models in CUDA. Biomedical Simulation, Lecture Notes in Computer Science 2008;5104(2008):49–58.

43. Sakashita T, Sando I. Postnatal development of the internal auditory canal studied by computer-aided three-dimensional reconstruction and measurement. Ann Otol Rhinol Laryngol 1995;104:469–75.

44. Sando I, Takahashi T. Stereophotography of computer-aided 3-dimensional reconstructions of the temporal bone structures. Otolaryngol Head Neck Surg 1996; 115(2); 811.

45. Sando I, Sudo M, Suzuki C. Three-dimensional reconstruction and measurement study of human eustachian tube structures: a hypothesis of eustachian tube function. Ann Otol Rhinol Laryngol 1998;107:547–54.

46. Takagi A, Sando I. Computer-aided three-dimensional reconstruction and measurements of the vestibular end-organs. Otolaryngol Head Neck Surg 1988;98(3):195–202.

47. Takagi A, Sando I. Computer-aided three-dimensional reconstruction: a method of measuring temporal bone structures including the length of the cochlea. Ann Otol Rhinol Laryngol 1989;98:515–22.

48. Yasumura S, Takahashi H, Sando I, et al. Facial nerve near the external auditory meatus in man: computer reconstruction study-preliminary report. Laryngoscope 1993;103:1043–7.

49. Sørensen MS, Dobrzeniecki AB, Larsen P, et al. The visible ear: a digital image library of the temporal bone. ORL J Otorhinolaryngol Relat Spec 2002;64(6):378–81.

50. Harada T, Ishii S, Tayama N. Three-dimensional reconstruction of the temporal bone from histological sections. Arch Otolaryngol Head Neck Surg 1988;114:1139–42.

51. Green JD Jr, Marion MS, Erikson BJ, et al. Three-dimensional reconstruction of the temporal bone. Laryngoscope 1990;100(1):1–4.

52. Kuppersmith RB, Johnston R, Moreau D, et al. Building a virtual reality temporal bone dissection simulator. Stud Health Technol Inform 1997;39:180–6.

53. Mason TP, Applebaum EL, Rasmussen M, et al. The virtual temporal bone. Stud Health Technol Inform 1998;50:346–52.
54. Vhp -NLM. 2010. Available at: http://www.nlm.nih.gov/research/visible/visible_human.html.
55. Volsky PG, Hughley BB, Peirce SM, et al. Construct validity of a simulator for myringotomy with ventilation tube insertion. Otolaryngol Head Neck Surg 2009;141: 603–8.
56. Serra L, Kockro R, Goh LC, et al. The DextroBeam: a stereoscopic presentation system for volumetric medical data. Proc. of Medicine Meets Virtual Reality 2002;10:478–84.
57. Agus M, Giachetti A, Gobbetti E, et al. Mastoidectomy simulation with combined visual and haptic feedback. Proc. of Medicine Meets Virtual Reality 2002;10:17–23.
58. Agus M, Giachetti A, Gobbetti E, et al. A haptic model of a bone-cutting burr. Proc. of Medicine Meets Virtual Reality 2003;11:4–10.
59. John NW, Thacker N, Pokric M, et al. An integrated simulator for surgery of the petrous bone. Proc. of Medicine Meets Virtual Reality 2001;9:21–4.
60. Pflesser B, Leuwer R, Tiede U, et al. Planning and rehearsal of surgical interventions in the volume model. Proc. of Medicine Meets Virtual Reality 2000;9:259–64.
61. Morris D, Sewell C, Barbagli F, et al. Visiohaptic simulation of bone surgery for training and evaluation. IEEE Trabs Comput Graph Appl 2006;26(6):48–57.
62. Sewell C, Morris D, Blevins NH, et al. Validating metrics for a mastoidectomy simulator. Proc. of Medicine Meets Virtual Reality 2007;15:421–6.
63. Sewell C, Morris D, Blevins NH, et al. Providing metrics and performance feedback in a surgical simulator. Comput Aided Surg 2008;13(2):62–81.
64. Wiet GJ, Stredney D, Kerwin T, et al. Dissemination/validation of virtual simulation temporal bone dissection: a project update [abstract]. Assoc Res Otolaryngol Annual Meeting Abstracts 2006;718.
65. Kerwin T, Shen HW, Stredney D. Enhancing realism of wet surfaces in temporal bone surgical simulation. IEEE Trans Vis Comput Graph 2009;15(5):747–58.
66. Available at: http://www.youtube.com/watch?v=Y_6finmrqao.
67. Stredney D, Wiet GJ, Bryan J, et al. Temporal bone dissection simulation: an update. Proc. of Medicine Meets Virtual Reality 2002;10:507–13.
68. Wiet GJ, Bryan J, Dodson E, et al. Virtual temporal bone dissection. Proc. of Medicine Meets Virtual Reality 2000;8:378–84.
69. Wiet GJ, Stredney D. Update on surgical simulation: the Ohio State University experience. Otolaryngol Clin North Am 2002;35(6):1283–8.
70. Kerwin T, Hittle B, Shen HW, et al. Anatomical volume visualization with weighted distance fields. Presented at The second Eurographics Workshop on Visual Computing for Biology and Medicine (VCBM). Leipzig, Germany: July 2, 2010.
71. Available at: http://www.youtube.com/watch?v=DViQuoPxycM&feature=channel.
72. McDonald S, Alderson D, Powles J. Assessment of ENT registrars using a virtual reality mastoid surgery simulator. J Laryngol Otol 2009;123:e14.
73. Zirkle M, Taplin MA, Anthony R, et al. Objective assessment of temporal bone drilling skills. Ann Otol Rhinol Laryngol 2007;116(11):793–8.
74. Jackson A, John NW, Thacker NA, et al. Developing a virtual reality environment in petrous bone surgery: a state-of-the-art review. Otol Neurotol 2002;23(2): 111–21.
75. Neri E, Sellari Franceschini S, Berrettini S, et al. IERAPSI project: Simulation of a can wall-up mastoidectomy. Comput Aided Surg 2006;11(2):99–102.

76. Sorensen MS, Mosegaard J, Trier P. The visible ear simulator: a public PC application for GPU-accelerated haptic 3D simulation of ear surgery based on the visible ear data. Otol Neurotol 2009;30(4):484–7.

77. Sowerby LJ, Rehal G, Husein M, et al. Development and face validity testing of a three-dimensional myringotomy simulator with haptic feedback. J Otolaryngol Head Neck Surg 2010;39(2):122–9.

78. Caversaccio M, Langlotz F, Nolte LP, et al. Impact of a self-developed planning and self-constructed navigation system on skull-base surgery: 10 years of experience. Acta Otolaryngol 2007;127(4):403–7.

79. Clijmans T, Gelaude F, Abeloos J, et al. Integration of application-specificity and automation in computer-aided pre-operative planning of mandibular reconstruction surgery. Int J CARS 2007;2:S226–235.

80. Xu X, Ping FY, Chen J, et al. [Application of computer aided design/computer aided manufactured techniques in mandible defect reconstruction]. Zhonghua Kou Qiang Yi Xue Za Zhi 2007;42(8):492–5 [in Chinese].

81. Leung R, Samy RN, Leach JL, et al. Radiographic anatomy of the infracochlear approach to the petrous apex for computer-assisted surgery. Otol Neurotol 2010;31(3):419–23.

82. Sessanna D, Stredney D, Hittle B, et al. Simulation of punch biopsies: a case study. Proc. of Medicine Meets Virtual Reality 2008;16:451–3.

83. Sparks J, Dupaix RB. Constitutive modeling of rate dependent stress-strain behavior of human liver tissue in blunt impact loading. Ann Biomed Eng 2008; 36:1883–92.

84. Stanford sinus surgery. Stanford; 2009. Available at: http://www.youtube.com/watch?v=KxpjiVDVo8Y.

85. Wiet GJ, Rastatter J, Bapna S, et al. Training otologic surgical skills through simulation – moving towards validation: a pilot study and lessons learned. J Grad Med Educ 2009;1(1):61–6.

Cell Phones in Telehealth and Otolaryngology

Jessica I. Kenyon, MA[a], Ronald Poropatich, MD[b],
Michael R. Holtel, MD[c],*

KEYWORDS

• Mobile health technologies • Remote monitoring
• Telemedicine • Remote data collection
• Cell phone health applications

Globally, cell telephones are among the most ubiquitous technologies today. A staggering 60% of the world's population owns a cellular telephone, a statistic surpassing even ownership of televisions.[1] Mobile technologies have become the platform of choice for consumers and industry. With 5.3 billion mobile subscribers as of 2010, its presence is so significant that it surpassed the number of people in the world with toothbrushes by twofold. With greater access to mobile telephones including rural areas, the potential of lowering information and transaction costs to deliver health care improves. Mobile technologies power the tablet or slate computer movement, which has expanded at a dramatic rate in the past few years. Coupled with this movement is the application store experience, which allows the user to personalize and customize mobile technologies for their specific needs. Paralleling this popularity, the use of cellular telephones in medicine is expanding. To date, there is a paucity of objective outcome data available on the efficacy of cell phones as an aid in telehealth, medicine in general, and otolaryngology specifically. Anecdotal data suggest, however, that although many applications of cell phone technology are quite simple, they are nevertheless effective in meaningful ways that can impact patient outcomes.

The healthcare community, which includes the military health system, now recognizes that mobile devices represent an enormous opportunity for healthcare outreach.

Views expressed in this article do not represent the US Army, Sharp Rees Stealy, or the University of Hawaii.

[a] US Army Telemedicine and Advanced Technology Research Center (TATRC), West Coast Satellite Office, US Army Medical Research and Materiel Command (USAMRMC), 4640 Admiralty Way, Suite 1030, Marina del Rey, CA 90292, USA

[b] US Army Telemedicine and Advanced Technology Research Center (TATRC), US Army Medical Research and Materiel Command (USAMRMC), 504 Scott Street, Fort Detrick, MD 21702, USA

[c] US Army Telemedicine and Advanced Technology Research Center (TATRC), US Army Medical Research and Materiel Command (USAMRMC), San Diego, CA 92106, USA

* Corresponding author. Sharp Rees Stealy, 10670 Wexford Street, San Diego, CA 92131.
E-mail address: mholtel@hawaii.edu

Otolaryngol Clin N Am 44 (2011) 1351–1358
doi:10.1016/j.otc.2011.08.013
0030-6665/11/$ – see front matter Published by Elsevier Inc.

Social networks, too, now go hand-in-hand with mobile devices. Statistics show that more people access social networks using the mobile World Wide Web than they do using desktop computers.[1] There are concerns using social networks because of the lack of confidentiality of these networks, but newer social networks, such as Google+, address some of these privacy concerns making them potentially more useful in medicine. There is some age disparity in the use of mobile technologies, but still overall mobile devices are the tool of choice for communication in the virtual sphere. As a result, cell phones represent a tool that can reach a very substantial patient population.

Strong evidence exists to suggest that mobile health technologies can help to bring about behavior change by impacting healthcare challenges, such as smoking cessation, diabetes, and appointment attendance.[2] Applications for cell phone platforms are emerging that enable clinical consultation, patient and provider education, research, biosurveillance, and disease management. Leveraging mobile devices in health care has been limited because of challenges in integrating their use in routine clinical practice and the security concerns of these devices on the commercial and military networks. Most applications have relied on mobile device primary function of communication via voice, short message service (SMS) text, and email. To deliver better value and improve access, healthcare organizations need to invest in commodity mobile technologies and modernize the clinical mobile experience that supports a variety of uses as a common service:

- Point of care
- Emergency response systems
- Human resources coordination, management, and supervision
- Mobile synchronous (voice) and asynchronous SMS telemedicine diagnostic and decision support to remote clinicians
- Clinician-focused, evidence-based decision support
- Pharmaceutical supply chain integrity
- Patient safety systems
- Clinical care and remote patient monitoring
- Health extension services
- Health services monitoring and reporting
- Health-related mLearning for the general public
- Training and continuing professional development for healthcare workers
- Health promotion and community mobilization
- Support of chronic conditions
- Remote data collection, such as industrial hygiene assessments
- Medication monitoring for dose adjustment and side effect documentation.

FEDERAL GOVERNMENT FUNDING TO ADVANCE MOBILE HEALTH

As mobile health use evolves from preclinical encounters (wellness tips; appointment reminders; and behavior change notices, such as smoking cessation) between the patient and the healthcare team, to clinical encounters (ie, medication change, subspecialty referrals) where treatment and management decisions are made, it is critical to document this encounter in the electronic health record (EHR). The Health Information Technology for Economic and Clinical Health (HITECH) Act of 2009 was established to accelerate the adoption of EHRs (meaningful use) and spur innovation in healthcare delivery by establishing financial incentives ($19–$27 billion) to practices and hospitals.[3] The HITECH Act is an aggressive and deliberate effort by the government to introduce health information technology into clinical settings with a deliberate goal of producing a safer, more efficient, more reliable, and more effective healthcare delivery system. Widespread adoption of EHRs is a prerequisite to widespread use of mobile health for clinical encounters. Complementing and further supporting HITECH, is the Affordable Care Act of 2010, which underscores the importance of health information technology in achieving goals related to health care quality and cost. This Act established the Center for Medicare & Medicaid Innovation to test innovations in care delivery and payments in diverse practices and will further potentially aid the widespread adoption of mobile health in clinical practice.

MOBILE DEVICES IN HEALTH CARE: A SURVEY OF CURRENT WORK

In telemedicine, and in particular, teleotolaryngology, cell phones are being used for some of the most fundamental capabilities, such as remote consultation.[4] Camera telephones have been used, for instance, to send photographs of nasal fractures to specialists for consultation.[5] Mobile telephones equipped with cameras have also enabled clinicians to transmit radiologic images for quick assessment in head and neck emergency situations.[6]

The availability and user acceptance of cell phones have allowed them to impact health care in ways that go well beyond traditional teleconsultation. Mobile health care using cell phones and other mobile technologies can be broken down into four key areas: (1) mobile health applications for patients, (2) remote data collection, (3) remote monitoring and diagnostics, and (4) decision support and mobile learning. A number of large-scale mobile health efforts are underway.

Mobile Health Applications for Patients

Txt2stop involved 5800 smokers from the United Kingdom in a randomized single-blinded study of smoking cessation SMS text messaging versus standard smoking cessation treatment and demonstrated a modest but statistically significant difference in smoking cessation in the SMS text group (cessation chemically verified at 6 months).[7] An earlier (2009) Cochrane review of mobile telephone–based smoking cessation studies had not shown a long-term difference.[8] Many medical systems offer the option of voice messages or SMS text messages as appointment reminders.

The US Military medical facilities have implemented programs that use personal cell phones to remind patients of appointments, to disseminate health and wellness information, and to gather important information from patients that can alert clinicians in real time to their status. At the Walter Reed Army Medical Center, cell phones are being studied as a tool for improving adherence to diabetes therapy.[9] The US Army's mCare provides secure SMS text messaging for patients, particularly targeting post-traumatic stress and traumatic brain injury patients. This program delivers appointment reminders to these patients, who often find the task of keeping multiple medical appointments challenging. In addition, mCare provides wellness information and disseminates general announcements pertinent to the patient. Initial data suggest that this very simple tool has had a positive impact on the military traumatic brain injury and posttraumatic stress patient population, mainly by increasing their likelihood of continuing and complying with treatment.[10] As part of its health diplomacy, the US Army has initiated efforts to offer a SMS texting program targeting public health (particularly pediatric and maternal–fetal care) to assist developing nations.[3] In the otolaryngology literature, use of text messages has reduced missed appointments at an outpatient clinic.[11]

In February 2010, the National Healthy Mothers Healthy Babies Coalition initiated the Text4baby program, a free mobile information service that provides health information to more than 131,000 pregnant women to promote maternal and child health.

Text4baby messages also tell women how to access public clinics and support services for prenatal and infant care.[12]

Remote Data Collection

Cell phones have evolved into tools for remote data collection, which can be especially useful in developing countries where a cellular infrastructure exists, even if other capabilities are lacking. Healthcare workers at the local level can upload health data by mobile device allowing disease surveillance, timely public health decisions, and feedback to the local healthcare worker via SMS text. The United Nation foundation global solutions Web site lists 15 active remote data collection projects. Examples include AIDS monitoring in Rwanda, malaria monitoring in Mozambique, a mobile-based primary healthcare management in India, and a community health information tracking system in the Philippines.[13] No specific examples for otolaryngology were available, but one could imagine remote hearing testing or data on head and neck cancer uploaded to a central database to provide an accurate measure of the disease burden with SMS text back to healthcare workers providing advice to manage that burden.

Remote Monitoring

Remote monitoring with mobile telephones and coupled sensors or wireless body area networks allows for objective physiologic measurements outside of the medical clinic with potential real-time feedback. The rapid growth in physiologic sensors, low-power integrated circuits, and wireless communication has enabled a new generation of wireless sensor networks that can be used for rehabilitation or early detection of medical conditions.[14] Objective mobile health monitoring will be further advanced through the integration of wireless communications with miniaturized biosensors that are either worn externally or implanted. Biosensors currently measure and track specific body physiologic parameters, such as electrocardiogram, temperature, heart rate, blood pressure, weight, breathing, blood sugar, and electroencephalogram waves. The most likely wireless communication, Bluetooth or ZigBee, will communicate with a mobile device, creating a body area network to represent the communications on, in, and near only the body. Captured physiologic data will be transmitted wirelessly from the sensors to a mobile device, which then transmits the data over the Internet or a wireless telecommunications system to a remote computer, monitoring system, concerned family member, or primary healthcare provider.

Challenges in full-scale implementation include interoperability of data across different wireless networks, security of data transfer to maintain HIPAA standards, sensor validation in variable power settings, and simplicity and ease of use of system design.

Although a wireless body area network can involve multiple sensors it can also be a simple as recording exercise data using a shoe-based GPS system, such as the Nike iPhone application to monitor the activity level for a weight loss program. Current efforts in otolaryngology have focused on balance. Researchers at the University of California Los Angeles's wireless health institute and the Massachusetts Institute of Technology have developed sensors incorporated into the insoles of patients' shoes that record balance and gait parameters. The Massachusetts Institute of Technology (through US Army-DARPA funding) has developed a foot strike power generation system that promises to supply power to the system once reliability issues are solved. The University of California Los Angeles insole effort (**Fig. 1**) is currently in its third-generation of insole that includes 40 pressure sensors and an accelerometer, and is actively undergoing clinical testing (Majid Sarrafzadeh, PhD, personal communication,

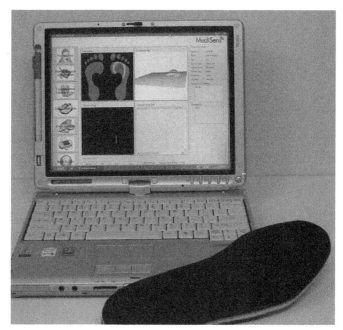

Fig. 1. MediSens balance insoles. (*Courtesy of* Majid Sarrafzadeh, PhD.)

2011). This technology provides an object measure for home vestibular therapy not currently available.

Remote Diagnostics

Examples of diagnostics with mobile devices include coupling a mobile telephone with a fluorescence microscope (**Fig. 2**) to aid in field diagnosis of disease,[15,16] an ultrasound machine for use in trauma,[17] or a glucometer for diabetes management.[18] Regarding diagnostics in otolaryngology, the ultrasound machine for trauma does not have the fidelity for most applications with the head and neck but the necessary fidelity will likely be available in the future. Several mobile telephone applications have been created for diagnostic audiologic testing, which has potential use for hearing screening.

Decision Support and Mobile Education

For decision support and education, popular medical applications include epocrates, Medscape, Reach MD, MicroMedix, *New England Journal of Medicine*, and various radiology tutorials. iResus, a smart telephone application, allows healthcare providers to perform better, more efficient cardiopulmonary resuscitation in a controlled randomized study.[19] A search for otolaryngology-specific decision support and education applications in the iPhone store did not reveal any results.

HEALTH CONCERNS WITH CELLULAR PHONES

Several articles have raised health concerns with the long-term use of cell phones in daily communications. There is no prospective study that demonstrates a definitive risk, but concerns have been raised about hearing loss, epithelial tumors of the parotid gland, and specific brain tumors.[20]

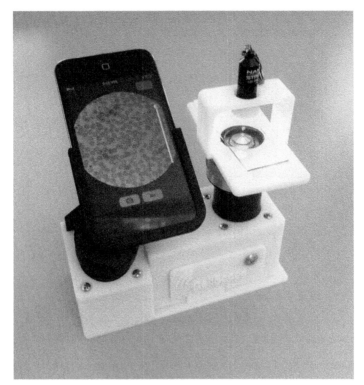

Fig. 2. Cell phone coupled to microscope. (*Courtesy of* Dan Flecher, PhD.)

CRITICAL CHALLENGES TO MOBILE HEALTH ADOPTION

There are numerous challenges to adopting mobile health in clinical practice.

- Integration of mobile applications with legacy information systems and EHRs currently is virtually nonexistent in 2011 and will be aided by the HITECH Act and federal funding. When fully implemented, how will mobile health impact on the busy provider who may already be suffering from excessive emails, telephone calls, and information overload? Management of mobile health data may require a health care team approach whereby clinicians are notified of clinical issues only after nonphysician providers have triaged the mobile health data.
- Technical challenges currently exist in support of a variety of handheld devices (eg, iPhone, Android, Blackberry) and a variety of network connections (eg, 802.11 wireless local area network/wi-fi, Bluetooth personal area network, wireless broadband wide area network, ultra wideband). These challenges will only be resolved when standards are adopted to facilitate data interoperability across networks and devices.
- Security, privacy, and confidentiality of patient data on the handheld device and during transmission remains an unresolved challenge with HIPAA-compliant "secure messaging" solutions now being developed commercially.
- The Food and Drug Administration is active in determining if medical data transmitted over a cellular network maintains the data fidelity generated from the

originating source (ie, electrocardiogram or fetal monitor). The potential impact is whether the commercial telephone used in mobile health is a mobile device or a medical device. This issue is evolving with commercial vendors working closely with the Food and Drug Administration.[21]

REFERENCES

1. Poropatich RK. TATRC's strategy for the research and development of mobile health applications. Presented at Mobile Health: The Use of Cell Phones for Healthcare Applications, a special session of the American Telemedicine Association Annual Meeting. San Antonio, May 15, 2010.
2. Krishna S, Boren SA, Balas EA. Healthcare via cell phones: a systematic review. Telemed J E Health 2009;15(3):231–40.
3. Kosaraju A, Barrigan CR, Poropatich RK, et al. Use of mobile phones as a tool for United States health diplomacy abroad. Telemed J E Health 2011;16(2):1–5.
4. Holtel MR, Burgess LP. Telemedicine in otolaryngology. Otolaryngol Clin North Am 2002;35:1263–81.
5. Moumoulidis I, Mani N, Patel H, et al. A novel use of photo messaging in the assessment of nasal fractures. J Telemed Telecare 2007;13(8):387–90.
6. Eze N, Lo S, Bray D, et al. The use of camera mobile phone to assess emergency ENT radiological investigations. Clin Otolaryngol 2005;30(3):230–3.
7. Free C, Knight R, Robertson S, et al. Smoking cessation support delivered via mobile phone text messaging (txt2stop): a single-blind, randomized trial. Lancet 2011;378(9785):49–55.
8. Whittaker R, Borland R, Bullen C, et al. Mobile phone-based interventions for smoking cessation. Cochrane Database Syst Rev 2009;4:CD006611.
9. Fonda S. A cell phone intervention for improving adherence to a diabetes therapy. Presented at Mobile Health: The Use of Cell Phones for Healthcare Applications, a special session of the American Telemedicine Association Annual Meeting. San Antonio, May 15, 2010.
10. Pavliscsak H. mCare: development, deployment, and evaluation of a mobile telephony-based patient secure messaging system. Presented at Mobile Health: The Use of Cell Phones for Healthcare Applications, a special session of the American Telemedicine Association Annual Meeting. San Antonio, May 15, 2010.
11. Geraghty M, Glynn F, Amin M, et al. Patient mobile telephone "text" reminder: a novel way to reduce non-attendance at the ENT out-patient clinic. J Laryngol Otol 2008;122(3):296–8.
12. Available at: http://www.cdc.gov/features/text4baby. Accessed August 14, 2011.
13. Available at: http://www.globalproblems-globalsolutionsfiles.org. Accessed August 14, 2011.
14. Ullah S, Higgins H, Braem B, et al. A comprehensive survey of wireless body area networks: on PHY, MAC, and network layers solutions. J Med Syst 2010. [Epub ahead of print].
15. Zhu H, Mavandadi S, Coskun AF, et al. Optofluidic fluorescent imaging cytometry on a cell phone. Anal Chem 2010. [Epub ahead of print].
16. Breslauer DN, Maamari RN, Switz NA, et al. Mobile phone based clinical microscopy for global health applications. PLoS One 2009;4(7):e6320.
17. McBeth PB, Hamilton T, Kirkpatrick AW. Cost-effective remote iPhone-teathered telementored trauma telesonography. J Trauma 2010;69(6):1597–9.

18. Carroll AE, DiMeglio LA, Stein S, et al. Using a cell phone-based glucose monitoring system for adolescent diabetes management. Diabetes Educ 2011;37(1): 59–66.

19. Low D, Clark N, Soar J, et al. A randomised control trial to determine if use of the iResus© application on a smart phone improves the performance of an advanced life support provider in a simulated medical emergency. Anaesthesia 2011;66(4):255–62.

20. Panda NK, Modi R, Munjal S, et al. Auditory changes in mobile users: is evidence forthcoming? Otolaryngol Head Neck Surg 2011;144(4):581–5.

21. Buntin MB, Burke MF, Hoaglin MC, et al. The benefits of health information technology: a review of the recent literature shows predominantly positive results. Health Aff (Millwood) 2011;30(3):464–71.

The Alaska Experience Using Store-and-Forward Telemedicine for ENT Care in Alaska

John Kokesh, MD[a],*, A. Stewart Ferguson, PhD[b],
Chris Patricoski, MD[b]

KEYWORDS

- Telehealth • Alaska Native Health System • Rural health clinics
- Remote health care • Health technology
- Remote ENT health care

Key Points: The ALASKA EXPERIENCE: TELEMEDICINE FOR ENT CARE IN ALASKA

- Store-and-forward telemedicine is well suited to the specialty of otolaryngology.

- Clinician involvement in selecting medical devices, creating protocols, and improving and modifying software are key to the success of a telemedicine program.

- Referring providers in Alaska believe that the use of telemedicine improves both clinical outcomes and patient satisfaction.

- The combination of high-quality images of the tympanic membrane and tympanometry data allows a diagnosis to be established in most telemedicine cases involving ear disease.

- Consultants using telemedicine should always have the options of recommending a traditional face-to-face encounter when appropriate care cannot be delivered solely through the telemedicine encounter.

- For facial trauma and facial plastics, review of images before seeing the patient has proved invaluable for consulting ear, nose, and throat (ENT) surgeons.

- A telemedicine system must have robust processes for initial and ongoing training, technical and clinical support, and technology assessment.

The authors have nothing to disclose.
[a] Alaska Native Medical Center, 4315 Diplomacy Drive, Anchorage, AK 99508, USA
[b] Alaska Native Tribal Health Consortium, 4000 Ambassador Drive, Anchorage, AK 99508, USA
* Corresponding author.
E-mail address: jkokesh@anthc.org

Otolaryngol Clin N Am 44 (2011) 1359–1374
doi:10.1016/j.otc.2011.08.010
0030-6665/11/$ – see front matter Published by Elsevier Inc.

Historically, Alaska Native and Canadian First Nations populations have been burdened with a high prevalence of otitis media and associated morbidity.[1–5] The incidence of ambulatory care visits related to otitis media for American Indian and Alaska Native children is twice that for all US infants, and the placement rate for tympanostomy tubes in these children younger than 5 years of age was 20 times higher in Alaska compared with the continental United States.[6] In addition, Alaska has an ongoing shortage of physicians, nurses, and allied health professionals, especially in rural and remote areas.[7,8] The ratio of physicians to population is less than the national average (2.05 MDs per 1000 population in Alaska vs 2.38 in the United States) and Alaska has the sixth lowest physician/population ratio in the nation.[9] The lack of access to medical specialty care, coupled with the high prevalence of ear disease, created a powerful motivator to develop innovative ways to extend the reach of physicians into rural Alaska.

The ear, nose, and throat (ENT) Department at the Alaska Native Medical Center (ANMC) initiated a telemedicine program in 1999 to help provide comprehensive ENT care.[10] The ENT Department resides within ANMC, a 150-bed, level II trauma center in Anchorage, Alaska, that provides specialty and tertiary care for the 130,000 Native Alaskans throughout the state. Most Alaska Natives live outside Anchorage in small communities and many live in remote villages only accessible by air travel. The ENT Department provides otolaryngology clinics at the Anchorage facility (daily) and at field clinics held at 6 regional hospitals (every 2–6 months). Patients living in rural Alaska need to travel to the regional hospital or Anchorage for the specialty clinic services. The need to service this remote population was the driving force to implement a better alternative for care delivery.

THE TECHNOLOGY

Store-and-forward telemedicine (electronic consultation) is well suited to augmenting otolaryngology services. Store-and-forward telemedicine is an asynchronous communication that allows the sender to take the necessary time to collect data from the patient and then send the case, which the consulting physician can later read and respond to when time is available. This method is convenient for the sender and receiver, and allows them to best use their clinical time. Store-and-forward telemedicine supports, replaces, or works with existing methods of communication. For example, scanned documents can replace faxes, and can be easier to find than paper faxes. Electronic data capture and keyboard entry removes the need for faxes and scans altogether. A store-and-forward case may remove the need for a telephone call.

Store-and-forward telemedicine (electronic consultation) has advantages compared with videoconferencing telemedicine, including that there is no need to synchronize the referring and consulting providers' time, no need to schedule a session using a videoconferencing network and bridge, low bandwidth requirements, minimal technical support needs, documentation of multimedia data for future reference, the potential for electronic data integration into electronic health records, and tracking of cases for time studies and administrative purposes.

The ENT Department uses the Alaska Federal Health Care Access Network (AFH-CAN) tConsult store-and-forward software developed by the Alaska Native Tribal Health Consortium (ANTHC) as the primary telemedicine communication tool. The department's physicians provided clinical advisory expertise during the software development process and served as one of the early deployment sites. The tConsult software is touch screen compatible, color coded for easy navigation, requires minimal training, and integrates with multiple biomedical devices such as the video otoscope, digital camera, self-administered screening audiometer, and tympanometer (**Fig. 1**). The software provides both a client-server model (for easy capture of data in clinics with poor or intermittent connectivity) and a Web-based interface for a patient-centric consultant display. The software supports secure client-to-server and server-to-server connectivity for a wide range of telecommunications infrastructure. There are a variety of software features that accommodate clinical workflow practices: cases can be sent to individuals or groups, consultants can be advertised locally or shared throughout an enterprise, and cases can be managed immediately or tagged for further work at a later time. Clinical guidelines for diagnosis, treatment, and triage can also be integrated into the software.

Cases are generated at remote village clinics or regional hospitals by health care providers using an AFHCAN telemedicine cart that includes tConsult software, biomedical peripherals, wireless network capability, and power management hardware (**Fig. 2**). In Alaska, most of these telemedicine carts are equipped with an audiometer, digital camera, dental camera, electrocardiogram, scanner, spirometer, stethoscope, tympanometer, video otoscope, and vital sign monitor. The ENT Department recognized the need early in the development process of the AFHCAN program for a high-quality video otoscope to visualize and capture images of the tympanic membrane (TM) and related structures. A comprehensive evaluation was conducted on the available video otoscopes, with the conclusion that the highest quality images could be obtained by using the AMD/Welch Allyn 300S Imaging and Illumination platform.[11] Continued use of this video otoscope led to best practices on image acquisition documented as a user's manual.[12] In time, it was recognized that some blurry images captured by providers were caused by improper focus, leading to the development of a focus tool used for prefocusing the equipment.[13]

The ENT Department also identified the need for tympanometry to be used in the field to supplement visualization of the TM. A review was conducted to identify an appropriate tympanometer that was easy to use and was reliable in the typical remote clinic setting.[14] This combined audiometer/tympanometer was integrated into the AFHCAN telemedicine cart and has since been a useful tool for ear and hearing assessment. Similar reviews were conducted to choose the most appropriate digital camera for dermatologic and facial imaging.

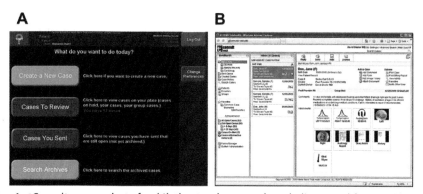

Fig. 1. tConsult screen shots for (*A*) the touch screen–based client used by providers to create cases, typically using this software on an AFHCAN cart, and (*B*) the Web client typically used by consultants to respond to cases. Note that all names and patient data are fictionalized.

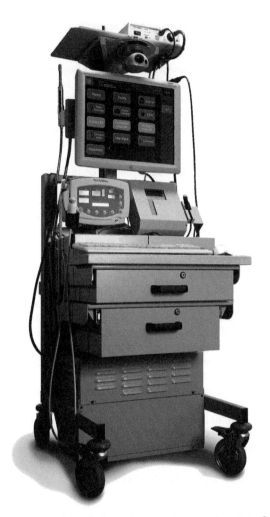

Fig. 2. The AFHCAN cart is a mobile platform that requires less than 0.4 m² of floor space in a small rural clinic, but provides the capacity to integrate a computer and touch screen with multiple biomedical peripherals such as an audiometer, digital camera, dental camera, electrocardiogram, scanner, spirometer, stethoscope, tympanometer, video otoscope and vital sign monitor. (*Courtesy of* AFHCAN, Anchorage, AK; with permission.)

The ENT Department continues to work closely with the ANTHC Telehealth Department to review and identify the best equipment for store-and-forward telemedicine applications. The need for a systematic, objective, and collaborative approach for selecting appropriate medical peripheral devices cannot be overemphasized because these tools become the eyes and ears for specialist operating at great distances from the patient.

VALIDATION AND CLINICAL BUY-IN

AFHCAN telemedicine carts were placed in all of the ENT Department examination rooms early in the project. Staff were introduced and trained on the telemedicine software and instructed on the use of the digital cameras and video otoscopes. Physicians initially used the equipment mostly for preoperative and postoperative images of the TMs and facial lesions. Later, the equipment was adapted for intranasal and laryngeal imaging. The carts were used as image acquisition stations for clinical documentation and archiving. The system was especially useful for patient education (eg, highlighting TM disorders and explaining the related middle ear problems). The staff quickly became experts on the hardware, software, and imaging techniques. They became comfortable receiving cases from the rural referring providers, could act as a resource for referring providers for matters related to image acquisition and case creation, and, most importantly, began to think creatively about the possible clinical applications of the technology. In retrospect, engaging the consultant providers in this way was a critical step in the development of the ENT telemedicine effort.

Although the benefits of video-otoscopy seemed obvious, there was little evidence to support its use as a means of providing clinical care. An initial study was conducted to determine whether TM images could be reliably used to substitute for in-person ENT care, comparing video-otoscopy with the in-person microscope examination for tympanostomy tube follow-up.[15] Forty patients who had tympanostomy tube placement in both ears were independently examined in person by 2 otolaryngologists and imaged locally by an expert telemedicine trainer/imager using a video otoscope and telemedicine software package. The 2 physicians later reviewed images at 6 and 12 weeks. For both physicians, the intraprovider concordance (agreement) between the in-person examination and the corresponding image review was high for each of the physical examination findings. The otolaryngologists were confident in their diagnosis, and confidence increased when cases with poor images were excluded (**Table 1**).

In a later study, TM imaging was performed by Community Health Aide/Practitioners (CHAP) on 35 patients in remote Alaska.[16] The patients were then flown to the regional facility where they were examined in person by 2 otolaryngologists. Images were later reviewed at 8 and 14 weeks. Similar to the first study, intraprovider concordance for physical examination findings was high (**Fig. 3**): tube in, 94% to 97% (κ = 0.89–0.94); tube patent, 94% to 97% (κ = 0.89–0.94); drainage, 90% to 96% (κ = 0.04–0.38); perforation, 90% to 96% (κ = 0.61–0.82); granulation, 97% to 100% (κ = 0.49–1.0); middle ear fluid, 88% to 96% (κ = 0.28–0.71); retracted, 83% to 91% (κ = 0.26–0.58). Although there were differences in the findings for the patients in person and later through images, this intraprovider agreement approximated the level of agreement found between 2 providers both seeing the patient in-person, which is the gold standard.

The overall conclusions drawn from these studies were that (1) the differences between viewing images and viewing TM in person were no different than the differences observed between 2 providers both viewing the patients in person, and (2) the results did not vary when images were taken in ideal conditions by an expert or when the images were taken by local providers in the remote village clinics.

USES

Uses for telehealth at ANMC have grown significantly since the first cases were received in March 2002 (**Fig. 4**). The ENT Department at ANMC has now responded to 9559 specialty telehealth consultation requests up to and including the most recent reporting date (12/31/2009). These cases were involved in the care delivery to 5751 Alaska Natives, and the involvement of more than 500 providers who created the telehealth cases. The most prevalent ICD9 primary diagnostic codes associated with the

Table 1
Evaluation question, confidence in diagnosis. Counts for each provider, and aggregate counts and percentages are shown for the responses to the Likert scale evaluation questions. Responses were provided during Review1 and Review2 with 1 response per physician per patient at T1 and again at T2 (total of 80 responses per provider)

		"Please Rate how Confident you are in the Diagnosis/Assessment Using Telemedicine in this Case"				
	[Blank]	1 = Not Confident at all	2	3 = Somewhat Confident	4	5 = Very Confident
Provider AA	0	5	7	14	33	21
Provider BB	1	2	4	10	23	40
Total	1 (1%)	7 (4%)	11 (7%)	24 (15%)	56 (35%)	61 (38%)

		"Please Rate how Confident you are in the Diagnosis/Assessment using Telemedicine in this Case"				
	[Blank]	1 = Not Confident at all	2	3 = Somewhat Confident	4	5 = Very Confident
Provider AA	0	1	4	12	33	21
Provider BB	2	0	2	5	22	40
TOTAL	2 (1%)	1 (1%)	6 (4%)	17 (12%)	55 (39%)	61 (43%)

Results only include images with adequate or better image quality.

From Patricoski C, Kokesh J, Ferguson S, et al. A comparison of in-person examination and video otoscope imaging for tympanostomy tube follow-up. Telemed J E Health 2003;9(4):331–44; with permission.

consultation requests were 384.2 (Perforation of tympanic membrane), 381.1 (Chronic serous otitis media), and 382.9 (Unspecified otitis media), accounting for approximately 33% of all cases.

The ENT Department has developed a process for responding to telehealth consultations in which a single provider has the daily responsibility to respond to that day's influx of telehealth consultation requests. The responsibility is rotated between providers, but this process allows the Department to turn around almost 75% of all telehealth cases in the same workday on which they are sent to ANMC from remote sites, and a 90% response rate within 24 hours (**Fig. 5**). This rapid turnaround time has continuously improved since 2002 because of process improvement within the ENT Department, and improved capabilities and features within the AFHCAN software to minimize the time involvement of ENT providers. The process is efficient enough to provide a 60-minute response rate to almost 30% of all cases, at times producing a specialty consultation response before the patient has left the remote clinic.

Providers that created cases to send to the ENT Department were asked to evaluate the system through a series of questions built into the AFHCAN software. These results, summarized in **Table 2**, indicate that more than 90% of providers sending consultation requests to the ENT Department believe that the system improves the quality of care for the patient and helps them communicate with the specialists, and find the software easy to use. A slightly smaller percentage, but still more than 5 of every 6 providers, believes that the system improves patient satisfaction and is satisfied and comfortable with the technology.

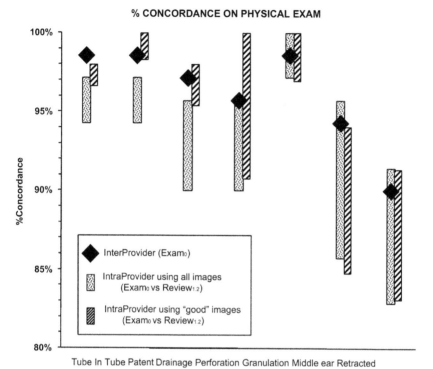

Fig. 3. Physical examination agreement from the second study, in which images were captured by providers at remote village clinics. The black diamonds indicate the percent concordance (agreement) between providers during the in-person examination (Exam0). The speckled bar indicates the range of concordance for individual otolaryngologists (intra-provider) between their descriptors at Exam0 and their descriptors during the image review (Review1 and Review2). The diagonally striped bars represent a similar minimum/maximum range for intraprovider concordance once ears were removed from consideration, for which the image sets were rated as having poor or very poor image quality. (*From* Kokesh J, Ferguson AS, Patricoski C, et al. Digital images for postsurgical follow-up of tympanostomy tubes in remote Alaska. Otolaryngol Head Neck Surg 2008;139:90; with permission.)

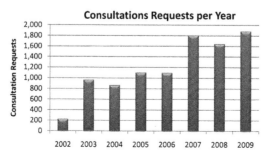

Fig. 4. Annual growth in requests for specialty telehealth consultation provided by the ENT Department at ANMC.

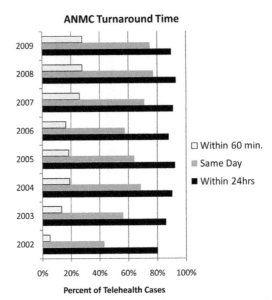

Fig. 5. Turnaround time for telehealth consultation request at the ENT Department at ANMC. Turnaround time is measured as the time from when a remote provider sends a telehealth case to ANMC until the ENT provider at ANMC responds to the case.

CLINICAL APPLICATIONS

The Alaska experience has shown that store-and-forward telemedicine using digital images has multiple applications in the diagnosis and treatment of ear disease. Care has been provided to large numbers of patients with otitis media, TM perforations, myringitis, otitis externa, and hearing loss. Store-and-forward telemedicine

Table 2
Responses to evaluation questions posed to providers that create telehealth consult requests that were sent to the ENT Department. In all cases, the initiating provider was asked to rate the statement using a Likert scale (with choices of Strongly Disagree, Disagree, Neutral, Agree or Strongly Agree). Providers were only asked a single question each time they created a telehealth case, each time the question being drawn from a pool of questions. The number of respondents to each statement is shown as (n = ...), and the percentage of responses that selected Agree or Strongly Agree is shown in the right column

"Please Rate the Following Statement":	Agree or Strongly Agree (%)
Telemedicine will improve the quality of care for this patient (n = 248)	93
Telemedicine helps me communicate with a doctor (n = 282)	92
The software is easy to use (n = 266)	91
I am comfortable creating a telemedicine case (n = 319)	87
Telemedicine improved patient satisfaction (n = 245)	87
I am satisfied with how the equipment worked (n = 241)	86
Telemedicine makes my job more fun (n = 284)	83
The telemedicine system played a role in educating this patient (n = 260)	67

has also proved useful for managing lesions of the oral cavity and oropharynx, laryngeal disorders, and problems related to facial plastics and facial trauma. In addition, this technology is being used increasingly for case management, facilitating triage, and helping to eliminate scheduling mistakes and loss of information.

Otitis Media

A good-quality image of the TM is often sufficient to diagnose acute or serous otitis media. Adequate focus, illumination, field of view, and color balancing before imaging are critically important. The validation studies referenced earlier indicated that images alone were, at times, insufficient when assessing problems related to middle ear pressure and TM mobility. An integrated tympanometer was added to the telemedicine cart and has proved to be a valuable addition, because the combination of images of the TM and tympanometry allows for diagnosis and treatment planning in most cases. Obstruction of the ear canal with cerumen, debris, or drainage prevents imaging in a minority of cases, and these need to be examined in a traditional face-to-face manner.

A recommendation for placement of pressure-equalizing tubes (PETs) rests on multiple factors, including the individual patient history, the appearance of the TM, audiologic and tympanometric data, and knowledge of current guidelines for when PETs are indicated. This information can be packaged into a store-and-forward telemedicine case for consideration by the consultant. In addition, through the collaborative efforts of clinicians and software developers, accepted clinical guidelines for PET placement have been incorporated into the software to seamlessly assist referring providers in following guidelines when referring patients. The interactive nature of store-and-forward telemedicine also makes it easy to request additional information on cases when necessary. Because the decision to place PETs often depends on the changes in clinical features with time (the appearance of a retracted TM, for example), the image archive that can be created as a result of serial store-and-forward cases on a given patient can be useful in monitoring for clinically relevant changes.

TM Perforations

We generally recommend repair of TM perforations for all otherwise healthy patients, beginning around age 6 years. Several factors influence the decision to offer elective tympanoplasty, including the patient history, the hearing and speech development status, the tympanometry results, and the appearance of both ears. In most cases, all of these factors can be effectively communicated and assessed using store-and-forward telemedicine. It is now routine in our practice to schedule elective tympanoplasty based on a store-and-forward telemedicine case, meeting the patient for the first time the day before surgery at the preoperative assessment and counseling appointment. A retrospective assessment of this practice (discussed later) indicates that both the operation needed and the operative time can be estimated as accurately from a store-and-forward telemedicine case as it can from a face-to-face encounter. Patient satisfaction with this practice has been high, with patients always having the option of foregoing telemedicine and choosing instead a traditional face-to-face consultation. Postoperative follow-up can also be readily accomplished using telemedicine, and patients from distant locations can be followed closely and for extended periods of time if necessary.

The experience using store-and-forward telemedicine for chronic ear disease brings up an important point: a clinician can decide at any point that a patient must be seen for an in-person examination, assessment, and counseling before a treatment decision is made. Even in these cases, the use of telemedicine provides background information and historical data for review before the patient encounter, making the in-person examination more focused and productive. In more complex cases in which imaging and ancillary studies are needed, arrangements for these can be made before the encounter.

Hearing Loss

Store-and-forward telemedicine is an effective tool for the assessment of previously undiagnosed hearing loss. The combination of history, images of the TM, audiogram, tympanometry, and, at times, otoacoustic emissions (OAEs) in almost all cases identifies conductive, neurosensory, or mixed hearing loss. For conductive losses, the cause is usually readily apparent and treatment can be planned. For neurosensory losses, those needing further evaluation can be identified and triaged, as in significant asymmetry. One of the most gratifying uses for store-and-forward telemedicine has been providing medical clearance for hearing aid fitting. In the past, many Native Alaskan elders in remote locations were unable to access hearing rehabilitation services and suffered from progressive hearing loss and its associated social isolation. Many are now assessed by a regional audiologist in their village, medically cleared using telemedicine, and subsequently fitted with a hearing aid, all within their village.

Not all remote regions in Alaska have the services of an audiologist, and a complaint of hearing loss cannot be addressed without some objective assessment of hearing. An automated audiometer has been integrated into the telemedicine cart and made available to clinics and providers who are unable to access the services of an audiologist. Although this device does not differentiate neurosensory from conductive losses, it does provide enough information to assist the consultant in making initial treatment and triage recommendations, and has proved to be a valuable addition to the AFHCAN system.

Facial Plastics and Reconstruction

Facial plastic surgeons have known for many years that standardized facial images are critical for documentation, planning, and follow-up of facial lesions and their treatment. Given the complex anatomy of the facial soft tissues and the difficulty that the referring provider often has in describing lesions, an image is probably the most important information that can be provided to the surgeon. We routinely require that images of facial lesions or deformities be sent for our review with the initial request for consultation. Whether the lesions are traumatic or neoplastic in nature, initial triage decisions and treatment planning can be completed before seeing the patient. For some traumatic soft tissue lesions, we have been able at times to advise the treating physician how best to close the wound, preventing the need for patient transfer. Readily available software paint programs can be used to mark images, detailing the specific steps for wound closure for the treating physician. When transfer is required because of the complexity of the lesion or the anticipated repair, the resources needed, such as operating room time, ancillary studies, or equipment, can all be arranged in advance. When image review is used in this way, the chance of finding that a facial lesion is more complex than had originally been described (too complex for an office procedure, for example) has been eliminated. For maxillofacial trauma, software integrating history, digital photography, and radiologic images has been found to be invaluable in triage and treatment planning before transfer of a remotely located patient.

Disorders of the Oral Cavity, Pharynx, and Larynx

Telemedicine is a useful tool for the diagnosis and management of diseases affecting the oral cavity, nasopharynx, pharynx, and larynx. In most cases using existing technology, a skill examiner can capture a high-quality image of a lesion at any of these sites. A portfolio of these images can be useful not only for establishing a diagnosis and treatment plan but also for following disease progression or treatment effect. For example, serial imaging of laryngeal carcinoma throughout treatment has been found by the author to greatly enhance patient education and compliance as well as disease documentation. Imaging the upper aerodigestive tract presents unique challenges. The medical devices needed to capture the highest quality images (dental camera for oral cavity and oropharynx and chip-in-tip flexible laryngoscope for hypopharynx and larynx) are expensive and, because of their high cost, not yet widely available. As these devices proliferate and high-quality images become more readily available, telemedicine applications will become more attractive for these anatomic regions. Capturing the dynamic function of the larynx is essential to diagnose many disorders. Although real-time video teleconferencing has been shown to be effective for this purpose, it requires the simultaneous availability of the patient and providers as well as significant bandwidth. Store-and-forward applications with the capability to asynchronously transfer short (up to 1 minute) video files may offer a more efficient solution. In addition, more intensive training and quality control is required if a nonotolaryngologist will be obtaining images of the nasopharynx or larynx.

AUDIOLOGIST ROLE

The audiologist can play a critical role in establishing a telemedicine program. Our program has had audiologists in the field who champion telemedicine by adopting the technology, expanding their clinical skills, communicating with the ENT Department, recruiting patients, creating cases, and following up with physician recommendations. Telemedicine allows audiologists to send images, clinical data, and hearing tests on both new and follow-up patients.

The partnership with audiologists proved successful in several ways. Regional ENT clinics were conducted every 2 months and clinics were so full that the typical wait time for scheduling a patient was 4 to 6 months. Regional audiologists began to use telemedicine to present referred patients to the consulting otolaryngologist. Appropriate triage and treatment decisions were made by the otolaryngologist; decisions that frequently obviated the need for the in-person encounter. This made in-person appointments available for other patients. A 16-year retrospective study (1992–2007) of new patient referrals to ENT specialty clinics at the Norton Sound Regional Hospital in Nome, Alaska, revealed that waiting times decreased from an average of 4.2 months before telemedicine to 2.9 months in the first 3 years with telemedicine, and then to 2.1 months in the next 3 years with telemedicine. Before telemedicine, 47% of new patient referrals waited 5 months or more to see an ENT specialist in person, but this decreased to 3% of all new patient referrals once telemedicine had been running for 6 years.[17]

An audiologist can also travel to underserved areas and deliver otolaryngology services if they are empowered with telemedicine technologies.[18] In a study conducted by ANMC and ANTHC, a traveling audiologist visited remote village clinics and created telemedicine cases that included clinical histories, images, audiograms, tympanograms, otoacoustic emission testing, and/or other documents. The otolaryngology consultants reviewed the cases and made treatment and triage recommendations. This system is ongoing for care delivery and has been in operation for the past 6.5 years, during which 67 trips have been made to 14 villages, providing 262 clinic service days. The mean patient encounter time is 32.7 minutes. Most patients received services for problems related to ears and hearing. Almost all patients had audiological testing by receiving tympanometry (90%), audiometry (68%), both (66%), or OAE testing (10%). Treatment plans or clinical intervention resulting from the audiology encounter and store-and-forward otolaryngology consultation are shown in **Fig. 6**. The 1987 patient encounters resulted in referral for surgery or special diagnostic testing (27%), referral for monitoring (26%), starting of medications (19%), referral to regional ENT clinic (13%), and referral to another specialty (6%). Approximately 26% of patients did not need to see the otolaryngologist and were triaged out of the specialty clinic.

The total cost to run this project was estimated at $175,000. Travel was avoided for 87% of encounters, resulting in travel cost savings in airfares of $697,090. These services were provided at a significantly lower cost and with fewer burdens to the patients compared with the standard referral system. This efficient care delivery model may be applicable to other specialties.

SURGICAL PLANNING

Telemedicine cases can be simple, moderate, or complicated. The decision process may result in the patient being reassured, treated, sent for additional testing, or referred to see the ENT specialist in person. Some telemedicine cases are direct referral cases for ENT surgery.

An analysis of a sampling of otologic cases led to the conclusion that store-and-forward telemedicine is as effective as in-person evaluation for planning elective ear surgeries such as tympanoplasty and mastoidectomy.[19] In this study, 45 ear surgeries recommended through telemedicine evaluation were compared with a matched set of 45 surgeries recommended through the standard in-person evaluation process. The surgeries included tympanoplasty with or without canalplasty, mastoidectomy, stapes surgery, and myringoplasty. Telemedicine and in-person evaluation accurately predicted the surgery 89% and 84% of the time, respectively. The average difference of actual time and estimated time for the surgical procedures performed was virtually indistinguishable (**Fig. 7**) and not statistically different between the 2 groups: 32 minutes for the telemedicine evaluation group and 35 minutes for the in-person evaluation group. Otologic surgeons are able to determine the needed surgery and required operative time as accurately as when patients were seen during a traditional in-person encounter.

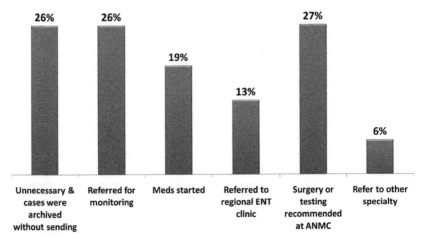

Fig. 6. Treatment plans. The clinical intervention resulting from the traveling audiologist using store-and-forward telemedicine with an otolaryngologist for 1987 patient encounters.

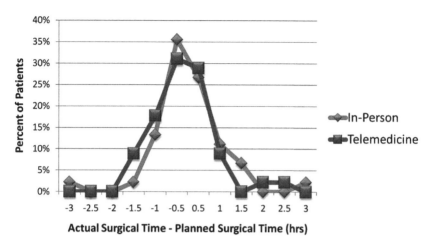

Fig. 7. A comparison of surgical time (actual surgical time minus estimated surgical time) for telemedicine and nontelemedicine (in-person) cases. Values in the right half of the plot represent cases that took longer than planned (42% of telemedicine cases and 47% of non-telemedicine in-person cases); values in the left half represent cases that took less time than planned (58% of telemedicine cases and 53% of nontelemedicine in-person cases). This histogram relies on a bin width of 30 minutes because operative times were estimated in increments of 30 minutes.

EDUCATIONAL CONTENT

One of the advantages of store-and-forward telemedicine is the automated collection of images and other multimedia. Recently, the ENT Department collected 28,000 otoscope and digital camera images from telemedicine cases. The best clinical images were reviewed, rated, and into a rich library collection. These images are now being used to develop educational content such as computer-based training for the clinical curricula of various health care providers.

TECHNOLOGY ASSESSMENT, TRAINING, AND SUPPORT

With more than 14,000 store-and-forward cases per year, the Alaska telemedicine system is mature and well integrated into the health delivery system. However, constant work is required to maintain and grow a telemedicine program. New medical devices with potential for use in telemedicine regularly enter the market. A formal process that uses clinical, technical, and software expertise to assess these products is essential; a poor technology decision can devastate a telemedicine program. Technology assessment is resource and knowledge intensive, and is best accomplished by dedicated centers. These centers can assist other programs with their technology decisions. Training and support are also critical ongoing needs. Provider turnover and changes in medical practice and technology are features of the health care environment. Without a robust training and support plan, even the best-conceived telemedicine plan deteriorates and fails as these factors evolve with time.

IMPACT OF THIS SYSTEM

The telemedicine system in Alaska is one of the world's most extensive networks, providing increased access, saved travel costs, and improved quality.[20] The AFHCAN has been in use since 2001 and has resulted in almost 70,000 store-and-forward clinical cases to date. With an ever-growing usage pattern now reaching 14,000 cases per year, this system is involved in care delivery to more than 12,000 Alaskans each year and is now considered an integral part of the day-to-day health care delivery system in the Alaska Tribal Health Systems (ATHS). More than 70% of all consultations prevent patients from having to travel to see specialists, resulting in statewide savings estimated at $3 million to $4 million annually in avoided patient travel costs (airfares). Specific to the ENT Department, 73% of all consultations prevent patient travel, and this has generally been consistent since the program was first adopted in 2002 (**Fig. 8**). A smaller, but significant, portion of telehealth cases (9% for ENT, 8% for all telehealth cases) cause patient travel, which is to be expected because disease states and various health issues are identified through telehealth, possibly at a much earlier and more easily treated stage in the disease state.

Continued usage of the system depends on many other factors, most notably the subsidies for connectivity provided through the Universal Service Fund subsidies for health care. Alaska also has a supportive reimbursement environment, with most insurers willing to reimburse for telehealth. It is still a struggle to show value to one segment of the health care industry when often the advantages are accrued by a different segment. For example, if payers do not cover travel for patients, the significant savings in patient travel for the health care system do not translate into direct benefits for that particular segment of the industry. This difficulty is perhaps the biggest challenge facing telehealth and the AFHCAN program, justifying the value of telehealth in an environment in which system impacts are less relevant than the direct bottom line impact for individual payer plans and programs.

Programs such as AFHCAN offer great promise for improving access to timely care for patients in remote communities across the Unites States and in many other

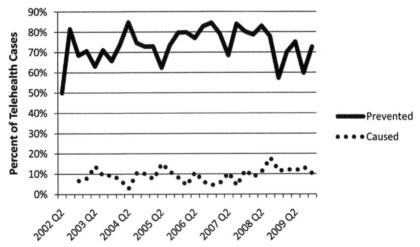

Fig. 8. Impact of ENT telehealth consultations on patient travel. The impact is measured by posing the following question to the consultants when responding to a telehealth case: "Did viewing this telemedicine case/image affect patient travel for diagnosis or treatment of this case (compared with a phone consult)?" Consultations select from one of the following options: "It had no effect on patient travel (same travel decision as phone consult)," "It caused patient travel," or "It prevented patient travel." The responses with the last 2 answers (caused and prevented) are shown in this figure as a percentage of all responses in each 3-month period.

countries. The success of these programs depends on many factors, perhaps the most important being relevance to the provider community that it serves. The single most important measure of the AFHCAN program is that clinicians not only continue to use it but more clinicians use it with more patients every year.

REFERENCES

1. Hamman C, Keeler F. Eye, ear, nose and throat infections in natives of Alaska. Northwest Med 1957;56:423.
2. The McGroth report: a documentation on the study and prevention of upper respiratory disease. Washington DC: State of Alaska, US Government Printing Office; 1962.
3. Baxter JD. Otitis media in Inuit children in the eastern Canadian Arctic—an overview—1968 to date. Int J Pediatr Otorhinolaryngol 1999;49(Suppl 1): S165–8.
4. Bruneau S, Ayukawa H, Proulx JF, et al. Longitudinal observations (1987-1997) on the prevalence of middle ear disease and associated risk factors among Inuit children of Inukjuak, Nunavik, Quebec, Canada. Int J Circumpolar Health 2001; 60(4):632–9.
5. Hodgins S. Health and well-being challenges in Nunavik: health conditions, determinants, and lines of action. Kuujjuaq (QC): Department of Public Health, Nunavik Regional Board of Health and Social Services; 1996.
6. Singleton RJ, Holman RC, Plant RL, et al. Otitis media outpatient visits and tympanostomy tube placement rates in young American Indian and Alaska Native children: what are the trends? Abstract in: 2nd International Meeting on Indigenous Child Health. Montreal, April 20–22, 2007.
7. Health Resources and Services Administration Web site. US Department of Health and Human Services; 2009. Available at: http://hpsafind.hrsa.gov/HPSASearch.aspx. Accessed March 1, 2009.
8. Alaska Center for Rural Health. Alaska's allied health workforce: a statewide assessment. Anchorage (AK): University of Anchorage; 2001.
9. Smart DR, Sellers J. Physician characteristics and distribution. 2008 edition. Chicago: American Medical Association; 2008.
10. Kokesh J, Ferguson AS, Patricoski C. Telehealth in Alaska: delivery of health care services from a specialist's perspective. Int J Circumpolar Health 2004;63: 387–400.
11. Ferguson AS. Video otoscope testing. Final report. Alaska Native Health Board. Anchorage (AK): University of Alaska Anchorage; 1998.
12. AFHCAN. User's manual. Video otoscope, AMD-300S (Welch Allyn/AMD) Document ID: Pub-112. Anchorage (AK): Alaska Native Tribal Health Consortium; 2006.
13. Patricoski C, Ferguson AS, Tooyak A. A focus tool as an aid to video-otoscopy. J Telemed Telecare 2003;9:303–5.
14. Patricoski C, Ferguson AS. Which tympanometer is optimal for an outpatient primary care setting? J Fam Pract 2006;55(11):946–52.
15. Patricoski C, Kokesh J, Ferguson S, et al. A comparison of in-person examination and video otoscope imaging for tympanostomy tube follow-up. Telemed J E Health 2003;9(4):331–44.
16. Kokesh J, Ferguson AS, Patricoski C, et al. Digital images for postsurgical follow-up of tympanostomy tubes in remote Alaska. Otolaryngol Head Neck Surg 2008; 139:87–93.

17. Norton Sound Health Corp, data on wait time reduction. (Report).
18. Kokesh J, Ferguson AS, Patricoski C, et al. Traveling an audiologist to provide otolaryngology care using store-and-forward telemedicine. Telemed J E Health 2009;15:758–63.
19. Kokesh J, Ferguson AS, Patricoski C. Pre-operative planning for ear surgery using store-and-forward telemedicine. Otolaryngol Head Neck Surg 2010; 143(2):253–7.
20. Hudson HE. Rural telemedicine: lessons from Alaska for developing regions. Telemed J E Health 2005;11(4):460–7.

Telemedicine: Licensing and Other Legal Issues

Gil Siegal, MD (TAU), LLB (TAU), SJD (UVa)[a,b,c,*]

KEYWORDS

- Telemedicine • EMR • Access to care • Licensure
- Informed consent • Malpractice • Confidentiality

The growth of information technology (IT) and telecommunications has created promising opportunities for better, faster, more accessible, barrier-free health care; what has become known as telemedicine (TM). Mastering technical issues or providing needed training remain important benchmarks for successful implementation of TM, but the legal issues constrain the progress of TM. As early as 2001, a report to the US Congress stated:

Key issues affecting the telemedicine and telehealth industry have remained the same over the past five years but their relative importance has changed with the advent of dramatic technology changes such as the wide spread adoption of the Internet.

These issues are[1]:

- Lack of reimbursement
- Legal issues
- Safety and standards
- Privacy, security and confidentiality
- Telecommunications infrastructure.

Except for the last point, these issues require legal resolution, a task most states have yet to resolve fruitfully, as well as professional associations (such as the World

Financial disclosure: no financial support was received for the preparation of this manuscript. The author has nothing to disclose.

[a] University of Virginia School of Law, 580 Massie Road, Charlottesville, VA 22903, USA
[b] Department of Oto-laryngology – Head & Neck Surgery, Tel Hashomer Hospital, Ramat Gan, Israel 52000
[c] Center for Health Law, Bioethics & Health Policy, Faculty of Law, 104 Zahal Street, Kiryat Ono College, Israel 55000
* Center for Health Law, Bioethics & Health Policy, Faculty of Law, 104 Zahal Street, Kiryat Ono, Israel 55000.
E-mail address: gil.siegal@ono.ac.il

Otolaryngol Clin N Am 44 (2011) 1375–1384
doi:10.1016/j.otc.2011.08.011
0030-6665/11/$ – see front matter © 2011 Elsevier Inc. All rights reserved.

Medical Association Statement on Accountability, Responsibilities, and Ethical Guidelines in the Practice of Telemedicine at the 51st World Medical Assembly, 1999).

This article identifies the key legal issues at stake, maps current legislation, and offers a forecast of needed legal/regulatory steps to expedite the dissemination of TM. The article is also aimed at readers with an interest in the business of TM[2] (either as providers or contemplating outsourcing of medical services such as diagnostics or imaging), as the feasibility of many TM projects depends on resolving legal issues. Topics not discussed in this article are e-commerce (such as e-prescription[3] and direct-to-consumer transactions), reimbursement, data protection and security (which is not unique to TM), and social networks.[4]

PREAMBLE

To assess the legal implications of TM, TM must first be defined. At least five states that have addressed TM in their statutes (Arizona, California, Georgia, Hawaii, and Oklahoma) use similar definitions. Telemedicine is "the practice of health care delivery, diagnosis, consultation and treatment and the transfer of medical data through interactive audio, video or data communications that occur in the physical presence of the patient, including audio or video communications sent to a health care provider for diagnostic or treatment consultation." (A.R.S. § 36-3601).

In the Report to Congress 2001, telemedicine refers to "the use of electronic communication and information technologies to provide or support clinical care at a distance." Telehealth is defined more broadly as "the use of electronic information and telecommunications technologies to support long-distance clinical health care, patient and professional health-related education, public health and health administration." Several teleinteractions and their legal status are shown in **Table 1**.

The practice of TM creates legal liabilities, starting with the overarching quandary of the legal right to practice TM, which is addressed later. Therefore, the answer to the question "Can I provide TM services?" depends on the type of activity. The construction of the medical activity defines the legal enabling requirements. For example, would it be (legally) wise to construct a consulting relationship rather than a treatment scheme? (The American Medical Association holds that this construction is unlikely to apply, and thus provide immunity, to regular, ongoing telemedicine links. See http://www.ama-assn.org/ama/pub/about-ama/our-people/member-groups-sections/young-physicians-section/advocacy-resources/physician-licensure-an-update-trends.shtml); or for an out-of-state provider to have a local physician as the on-the-ground, in-state anchor

Table 1 Some digital interactions and their legal status		
Type	**Is It TM?**	**Legal Liability: Establishing a Duty of Care[a]**
Email/SMS	Probably	Yes
Web site	No	Probably not
Fax	No	Yes/probably
Telesurgery	Yes	Yes
Teleradiology	Yes	Yes (either directly or by vicarious liability)[b]
Telemonitoring	Yes	Yes
Social networks (eg, Facebook)	No	No (except for confidentiality)

[a] It is impossible to survey all states' laws. This tabulation should be used only as a preliminary benchmark, because state-to-state variation is inevitable.
[b] See text.

that initiates and has ultimate authority over the patient? (FL Statutes–Title XXXII Regulation of Professions and Occupations Section 458.3255: "Only a physician licensed in this state or otherwise authorized to practice medicine in this state may order, from a person located outside this state, electronic-communications diagnostic-imaging or treatment services for a person located in this state.") Most states allow singular/infrequent interactions, and usually exempt consultations that are not compensated (eg, Hawaii, Colorado, and California allow significant consulting exceptions. In Alabama: "The 'irregular or infrequent' practice of medicine across state lines is deemed to occur if such practice occurs less than 10 times in a calendar year or involves fewer than 10 patients in a calendar year or comprises less than 1% of the physician's diagnostic or therapeutic practice"). Hence, you may be (legally) comfortable to render your medical opinion in peer consultation, but not to run a medical business without having to adhere to current licensure requirements in all states.

Licensure

The practice of medicine requires a license, a requirement based on the need to protect the public health from the practice of medicine by unqualified providers, as well as to protect the interests of the medical guild.[5] In most countries, practicing medicine without a valid license is a criminal offense. Some states or countries forbid the practice of medicine in another jurisdiction without a proper license in that second state, and disciplinary measures (including revocation of license) may ensue. In the United States, licensure has been a states' prerogative, and restrictive statutory licensure requirements for practicing medicine across state lines have been subject to growing criticism. It is hard to justify, based on public safety, why local requirements for a California license would be insufficient for practicing medicine in Colorado; citizens in both states should be similarly protected from the unqualified practice of medicine. This notion has been reflected in the Federation of State Medical Boards Special Committee on License Portability, 2002, recommending that state medical boards develop and use an expedited licensure by endorsement process to facilitate multistate practice.[6] Border-free TM provides another powerful reason to question this parochial segregation, and to call for a more uniform licensure process/requirement. By current (obsolete) understanding, a physician is considered to be practicing medicine in the state where the patient is located (by convention, originating site), which is hard to accept: because patients may travel to any state or country to be treated[7] at their sole discretion; why can they not travel electronically (being much more efficient, saving money, time, or the environment), thereby creating a legal way to allow TM according to the location of the treating professional? This plea has been heard in Europe, where a new, approved directive on cross-border health care (Directive on Cross-border Health Care - COM(2008)414) requires all states to create legislation that allow patients to receive health care in another member state and be reimbursed to the level of costs that would have been assumed by the member state of affiliation if this health care had been provided on its territory (although states may limit this for overriding reasons of general interest). Member states may introduce a system of prior authorization to manage the possible outflow of patients; however, it is limited to health care that is subject to planning requirements. Examples include hospital care; highly specialized and cost-intensive care, especially risky care; or health care that could raise serious concerns about quality or safety.

Current and Needed (Constructive) Licensure Practices

After almost 2 decades of attempts to ease the licensure uncertainty, not enough has been ascertained. A survey of states' licensure statutes reveals that most states still adhere to full, unrestricted licensure requirements for allowing the practice of medicine across state lines. However, there is a trend toward accepting the borderless nature of TM. To date, approximately 10 states (Alabama, California, Minnesota, Montana, Nevada, New Mexico, Ohio, Oregon, Tennessee, and Texas. Based on the Center for Telehealth and E-Health Law Report. Available at http://www.telehealthlawcenter.org/?c=118. Accessed July 19, 2010) have adopted some version of a limited/special purpose licensure, which allows practitioners to obtain a limited license for the delivery of specific health services in particular circumstances, which is suitable for the TM model. Practitioners are required to maintain a full and unrestricted license in at least 1 state, while practicing TM in others. For example, Montana created a telemedicine license that authorizes an out-of-state physician to practice telemedicine only in the specialty in which the physician is board certified. A telemedicine license authorizes an out-of-state physician to practice only telemedicine.

Another option that may assist fruitful dissemination of TM is a border-free TM national system that would issue a license based on universal standards for the practice of health care in the United States.[8] This does not necessarily preempt states' sovereignty, but represents a national agreement to be implemented by each state. The logistics would require sensible solutions (eg, how data would be collected and processed; setting standards of education, qualification, and training; disciplinary measures), but some progress has already been made, such as the establishment of the National Practitioner Data Bank,[9] the acceptability of Joint Commission on Accreditation of Healthcare Organizations (JCAHO; now The Joint Commission [JC]) as a national standard for medicine and practices, or the expanding reach of the US Food and Drug Administration (FDA) on health issues. In particular, in 2001, JCAHO introduced standards for institutional credentialing of TM providers. By these standards, a physician credentialed in any JCAHO facility would be permitted to provide TM services in another JCAHO facility (the JC rules allowed the facility where the patient is being treated to credential the distant treating physician in 2 ways: (1) the treating facility could fully credential the physician based on their own facility's standards; or (2) the treating facility could accept the credentials of the treating physician because the remote institution is JC certified. However, in 2009, CMS required that only option 1 remains valid. JCAHO announced that a final decision is still pending). A stronger version would attempt a federal licensure system that would preempt state licensure laws, issuing one license that would be valid throughout the United States.[10]

Another, less ambitious option, is for state boards to award licenses to professionals in other states with equal standards (endorsement). To have their licenses endorsed by another states, professionals need to apply for a license by endorsement from each state in which they seek to practice. However, because states may require additional qualifications or documentation before endorsing a license issued by another state, endorsement can be time consuming and expensive for a multistate practitioner in TM. To address part of this difficulty, a licensure system based on reciprocity requires the authorities (rather than individual practitioners) of each state to reach agreements to recognize licenses issued by the other state/s (bilateral or multilateral) without a further review of individual credentials. A license valid in one state would allow the practice of medicine in all other states with which such agreements exist; but notification or registration might still be needed. Such a requirement may be waived by mutual recognition, in which a state's licensing authority legally accepts the licensure of another state without further action. The nurse licensure compact, legally accepted in 24 states, is based on this model, and should be more vigorously studied.[11]

The most sensible and productive solution to TM licensure would be electronic patient transfer,[7,12] viewing TM as being rendered at the location of the physician, the distant site. JCAHO (revising its credential policy), opted that practitioners who render care using live/interactive systems are subject to credentialing and privileging at the distant site (where the consultant is located) when they are providing direct care to the patient. However, CMS has required a change of this resolution, requiring institutions to establish independently the credentials of remote TM practitioners. A final rule is expected by June 2011. Other solutions presented here subscribe to the notion that leaving things as they are is unacceptable, because the interests of patients (eg, where specialists are scarce), providers (eg, when they can offer better or more efficient care), and the health system at large (containing the rising costs and decreased availability) are not adequately served.[13] Moreover, scholars have argued that states' current legal barriers to TM are unconstitutional.[14] Attempting to circumvent current licensure by regarding all TM interactions as recommendations/consultation has several disadvantages: it probably will not pass legal scrutiny in most states' courts; it requires a local referring physician who keeps full authority and legal responsibility over the patient (Hawaii, Colorado, and California allow significant consulting exceptions); it restricts patients' autonomy in interacting with physicians at their convenience and choice; and it prevents a productive, cost-effective business model with an inhibitory effect on the uptake of TM.

Assuming that licensure issues have been resolved, or that TM is practiced within a state's borders (where no additional licensure for TM is needed), other legal issues emerge. For example, provider authentication remains a challenge.[15,16] TM should not be restricted on these grounds, because authentication requirements are shared by all IT-based modern enterprises (such as banking, credit, e-learning), and have been reasonably resolved. Therefore, TM should not be treated differently and available cyber-tech solutions should be used. Responsibility for assuring and protecting authentication is, and should be, the responsibility of the institution that provides the medical service, and appropriate regulations should be instituted and monitored (eg, passwords, event log/access archive, log-in log). In contrast, authentication in cyberspace is more problematic. Attempts to regulate cyberspace have proved futile in most cases (eg, pharmaceutical, direct-to-consumer genetic tests), and the responsibility should be shifted to consumers, expecting them to use only credible sources. Consumers should be empowered by information on the hazards of receiving medical care or consultation from nonaffiliated practitioners, as well as listing flawed sources/sites (as with travel warnings).

A final related question refers to choice of venue and law: if there is a multistate or multinationality TM interaction, which court should have jurisdiction, and what legal norms should be used?[17] Because TM will undeniably create legal disputes, such as claims of malpractice, this issue must be proactively determined. A thorough exposition of choice-of-law is beyond the scope of this article because it requires a case-by-case determination and can be found elsewhere.[18] However, most uncertainties can be resolved by binding (international) arbitration, as is commonly practiced by multinational commercial interactions (a result of the successful United Nations Convention on Recognition and Enforcement of Foreign Arbitral Awards, 1958, also known as the New York Convention).[19]

Legal Aspects Stemming from a Patient-Provider Relationship

Phase II questions (ie, beyond who may practice TM and where), target the legal implications of using TM to diagnose or treat patients. These liabilities stem from a patient-provider relationship (PPR), and are derived from tort doctrines and recognized professional liabilities, providing ample case law and statutes from which to infer.[20,21]

TM interactions are conducted in different models. One scenario involves a direct provider-to-patient interaction (also called the direct patient care model), such as in telemonitoring or telepsychiatry. A different model stipulates the presence of another provider at the originating site (also called the provider-to-provider consulting model), customarily practiced in ear, nose, and throat teleconsultation or telesurgery. The latter model places ultimate authority (and thus responsibility) on the provider at the originating site. Another model is devoid of patient presence altogether (eg, teleradiology). Such different modus operandi have important legal implications in creating binding PPR. Thus, the notion that all telemedicine is the same should be rejected and, within each TM interaction, the relevant components that can affect legal responsibilities and liabilities should be identified.

Informed Consent

Informed consent (IC) is a pivotal ethicolegal requirement. In TM, consent would be needed for 2 main reasons. The first is consent to the medical interaction itself (eg, diagnosis, treatment, monitoring), and the second refers to the transmission of medical and personal information via digital media, thereby sharing it with other providers and possibly (though not necessarily) storing it elsewhere.[22] The first requires deliberation regarding consent to medical treatment based on procedures, benefits, and risks; the latter refers to informational risks: privacy and confidentiality.

Legal advice concerning liabilities for IC in TM must clarify whether a particular TM interaction is different than its non-TM counterpart. For example, consent to a telesurgery procedure involves all the risks of the traditional procedure with additional risks (for example, failure of communication lines, or a need to convert a teleprocedure to a traditional one, perhaps by a different practitioner). As a result, the batch of information necessary for IC must be expanded to incorporate the unique features of TM. Professional bodies such as the AAO-HNS and their legal advisors should evaluate all TM interactions and clearly define the set of information required for valid IC, and should not leave it to the discretion of individual practitioners and the injudiciousness of juries in court.

A separate question relates to the identity of the provider responsible for obtaining consent from the patient. For example, in California, only a state-licensed physician can establish PPR. Thus, "[T]he health care practitioner who has ultimate authority over the care or primary diagnosis of the patient shall obtain verbal and written informed consent from the patient…" (Cal. Telemedicine Dev. Act 1996). Therefore, prime liability rests on the physician at the originating site. If a state allows out-of-state practitioners to diagnose or treat patients, I advocate that both physicians (at originating and distant sites) assure and document valid IC, preferably by a signed form. In a direct patient care model, the provider is responsible for valid IC.

Documentation of IC remains essential, and many information technologies are available to record and archive ICs for future contentions. All involved parties (especially in multinational interactions) should verify the accuracy and adequacy of the IC process, and maintain access to the signed IC forms for future reference. The new platforms of Dialog Medical's iMedConsent[23] or similar international companies enable providers to obtain standardized, automatic, computerized IC to manage legal risks and to improve patients' education.

Data protection and confidentiality are well-known concerns in TM, but have already received attention as a result of HIPAA (the Health Insurance Portability and Accountability Act of 1996, P.L.104–191)[24,25] and also the development of electronic health records (EHR).[26,27] Medical data might be transferred to distant sites in several situations. In teleradiology, imaging studies are transferred, whereas, in teleconsultation, entire medical records could be shared with others. Telesurgery or telepsychiatry would create a live video file that can be stored, copied, and transmitted. All these cases involve informational risks that must be contained and to which patients need to consent.[28] Some of these risks are not adequately met by current practices. Institutions and practitioners who outsource diagnostic services to out-of-state or to foreign countries rarely share this fact with their patients.[19,29] Although understandable from a prestige perspective or a business point-of-view, this practice raises serious concerns about patients' consent to such data transformation.[25]

Involving consultants in medical care requires providers to be transparent about their identity and qualifications, and to provide patients with binding assurances about record keeping, confidentiality, and the possibility of future access to their files (fair information practices). Patients must be given the opportunity to decline such transfers. As with legal advice, when applicable, institutions should attempt to make transferred medical records anonymous (for example, by using one-way codes) because the identity of the patient is not material to diagnosing a pathology slide or reading magnetic resonance imaging. In this case, most legal concerns are alleviated, because unidentified medical information (removing identifiers such as names, addresses, birth or hospital discharge dates, telephone or fax numbers, email addresses, social security numbers, medical record or health plan account numbers, or Internet Protocol [IP] address numbers) is not subject to the stringent regulation mentioned.

MEDICAL MALPRACTICE, STANDARDS, AND GUIDELINES

The American health system has been profoundly affected by medical malpractice litigation, resulting in an insurance coverage crisis, costly defensive medicine, and a less-than-adequate effort to improve patients' safety. It is difficult to predict the impact of TM on this situation, although, after more than a decade of practice (although scarce), no notable changes have been documented. Assuming a greater proportion of TM in the health care arena, several questions require resolution. What constitutes malpractice in TM? Should TM malpractice cases be treated differently by the courts? Are TM practices covered by current malpractice insurance policies, and would TM lead to another increase in costs?

To invoke malpractice, a plaintiff must establish that the provider has breached the duty of care owed to the patient (based on legally binding PPR) by performing at less than the standard of care expected from a reasonable professional in the same circumstances; a breach that directly brought about the injuries (causation).[30] Delineating the standard of care in TM is still in its early stages; however, this is only a matter of time. Thus, professionals should actively seek to canvas the standard of care in their respective specialties within the TM domain by producing comprehensive standards and guidelines. For example, the American Telemedicine Association's Core Standards for Telemedicine Operations[31]; the American Academy of Dermatology's minimal pixel resolution and connection speed standards[32]; the American College of Radiology Standards for Teleradiology[33]; or the standards for videoconferencing telemental health provisions.[34]

To date, there has been no court ruling on TM's standard of care, so it must be assumed that traditional malpractice precedents will serve TM cases, until new case law emerges. This assumption, in turn, requires reasonable care in medical history taking, using appropriate diagnostics, reaching a diagnosis based on adequate deferential diagnosis, choosing and providing accurate treatment in a reasonable manner, appropriate follow-up, and timely intervention if the need arises.

Regarding coverage, most policies exclude unlicensed activity. Therefore, practitioners must ascertain their coverage status (including licensure) before engaging in TM activity (with the exception of infrequent, not-for-profit teleconsultation). In 2007, the American Telemedicine Association endorsed a special insurance policy (TelMed, offered by The Campania Group) that provides clarification on the part of providers and guarantees full malpractice coverage. Other dedicated insurance products are available, and thus coverage issues should not halt the proliferation of TM if the policies clearly and unambiguously provide coverage for the specific TM activity being practiced.

CONCLUDING REMARKS

The author firmly supports the continuous progress of TM. The legal obstacles are numerous but not insurmountable, and more work needs to be done in adapting medical ethics and law to the digital era. Cyberspace has become important, and health care must keep pace with its development. Providers, the public, and policymakers should collaborate to enable improved prognosis and more rapid materialization of TM capabilities, as recently promulgated by the American Recovery and Reinvestment Act of 2009.

However, progress is contingent on removing barriers, of which the most pressing is the licensure impediment, to provide vital legal assurance for practitioners and investors. The most obvious breakthrough is electronic patient transfer. Accessibility should be incorporated in the promotion of TM, assuring that technological advancements are available to all. Special adjustments might be needed for people with disabilities (especially sensorineural deficits) or individuals without sufficient IT literacy.

Equipped with legal insights, physicians and entrepreneurs should reap the benefits of IT, contain risks, and achieve enhanced, accessible, and more efficient medical care. TM has a promising future and legal resolutions must be found.

REFERENCES

1. 2001 Report to US Congress on telemedicine. Available at: http://www.hrsa.gov/telehealth/pubs/report2001.htm. Accessed July 19, 2010.
2. A 2004 federal report estimated (at that time) a $380 million telemedicine market, with projected annual growth rates of 15% to 20%. See US Office of Technology Policy. Innovation, demand, and investment in telehealth. Washington, DC: Department of Commerce; February 2004 [cited in Singh SN, Wachter RM. Perspectives on medical outsourcing and telemedicine—rough edges in a flat world? N Eng J Med 2008;358:1622–7].
3. Holzhauser v. State Med. Bd., No. 06AP-1031, 2007 WL 5003 (Ohio Ct. App. Sept. 25, 2007). Golob v. Arizona Medical Bd. of State, 176 P.3d 703 (Ariz. Ct. App. 2008). In re Div. of Mental Health Servs., No. A-2966–07T2, 2009 N.J. Super. Unpub. LEXIS 1573 (App.Div. June 17, 2009).
4. Terry NP. Physician and patients who "friend or tweet": constructing a legal framework for social networking in a highly regulated domain. Indiana Law Rev 2010; 43:266.
5. See American Medical Association, Physician Licensure: an update of trends. Available at: http://www.ama-assn.org/ama/pub/about-ama/our-people/member-groups-sections/young-physicians-section/advocacy-resources/physician-licensure-an-update-trends.shtml. Accessed July 19, 2010. An up-to-date compilation of

states' regulation and licensure requirements in respect to TM. Available at: http://www.telehealthlawcenter.org/?c=118. Accessed July 19, 2010.

6. Available at: http://www.fsmb.org/pdf/2002_grpol_License_Portability.pdf. Accessed July 19, 2010.

7. Milstein A, Smith M. America's new refugees — seeking affordable surgery offshore. N Engl J Med 2006;355:1637–40.

8. For a legal analysis of federalism, Congress's powers and states' sovereignty see United States v. Lopez, 514 U.S. 549 (1995).

9. 401–432 of the Health Care Quality Improvement Act of 1986, Pub. L. 99–660, 100 Stat. 3784–3794, as amended by section 402 of Pub. L. 100–177, 101 Stat. 1007–1008 (42 U.S.C. 11101–11152). Available at: http://www.npdb-hipdb.hrsa.gov/legislation.html. Accessed July 19, 2010.

10. Department of Commerce. Report to Congress on Telemedicine (official document on file with author). 1997.

11. For the complete list of those 24 states. Available at: https://www.ncsbn.org/158.htm. Accessed July 19, 2010.

12. Burkett L. Medical tourism. Concerns, benefits, and the American legal perspective. J Leg Med 2007;28:223–45.

13. Venable SS. A call to action: Georgia must adopt new standard of care, licensure, reimbursement, and privacy laws for telemedicine. Emory Law J 2005;54:1183.

14. Gupta A, Sao D. The unconstitutionality of current legal barriers to telemedicine in the US: analysis and future directions of its relationship to national and international health care reform. 2010. Available at: http://works.bepress.com/deth_sao/2. Accessed July 19, 2010.

15. Perminov V, Antciperov V, Nikitov D, et al. Preventing unauthorized access to user accounts in a telemedicine consultation system. J Comm Tech Electron 2009;54:1319–21.

16. Bellazzi R, Montani S, Riva A, et al. Web-based telemedicine systems for home-care: technical issues and experiences. Comput Methods Programs Biomed 2001;64:175–87.

17. Dickens BM, Cook RJ. Legal and ethical issues in telemedicine and robotics. Int J Gynaecol Obstet 2006;94:73–8.

18. Clifford RD. Computer and cyber law: cases and materials. Durham (NC): Carolina Academic Press Law Casebook Series; 1999.

19. Zawadski P. International outsourcing plus inexpensive, quality healthcare: binding arbitration makes this telemedical dream a reality. Health Matrix Clevel 2008;18:137–79.

20. Blum JD. Internet medicine and the evolving legal status of the physician-patient relationship. J Leg Med 2003;24:413–55.

21. Derse AR, Miller TE. Net effect: professional and ethical challenges of medicine online. Camb Q Healthc Ethics 2008;17:453–64.

22. Goldstein MM. Health information technology and the idea of informed consent. J Law Med Ethics 2010;38:27–35.

23. Available at: http://www.dialogmedical.com/default.htm. Accessed July 19, 2010.

24. 42 USCA § 1320d-2.

25. Annas GJ. HIPAA regulations - a new era of medical-record privacy? N Engl J Med 2003;348:1486–90.

26. See Health Information Security and Privacy Collaboration (HISPC), initiated by the Department of HHS. Available at: http://healthit.hhs.gov/portal/server.pt?open=512&objID=1240&parentname=CommunityPage&parentid=2&mode=2. Accessed July 19, 2010.

27. Hodge JG, Gostin LO, Jacobson PD. Legal issues concerning electronic health information: privacy, quality, and liability. JAMA 1999;282:1466–71.

28. Recently, international standards have been developed by ISO. See ISO/TS 21547:2010, Health informatics – Security requirements for archiving of electronic health records – Principles; ISO/TR 21548:2010, Health informatics – Security requirements for archiving of electronic health records – Guidelines. Available at: http://www.iso.org/iso/catalogue_detail?csnumber=44479. Accessed July 19, 2010.

29. McLean TR. The future of telemedicine & its Faustian reliance on regulatory trade barriers for protection health matrix. J Law Med 2006;16:443–510.

30. A friendly text from the AAO-HNS Professional Liability Committee: The Professional Liability Handbook is available at: www.entnet.org/Practice/loader.cfm?csModule=security%2fgetfile&pageid=11105. Accessed July 19, 2010.

31. Available at: http://www.americantelemed.org/files/public/standards/CoreStandards_withCOVER.pdf. Accessed July 19, 2010.

32. Available at: http://www.aad.org/forms/policies/Uploads/PS/PS-Telemedicine%206-15-07.pdf. Accessed July 19, 2010.

33. Available at: www.acr.org/SecondaryMainMenuCategories/quality_safety/guidelines/med_phys/electronic_practice.aspx. Accessed July 19, 2010.

34. Available at: http://www.americantelemed.org/files/public/standards/PracticeGuidelinesforVideoconferencing-Based%20TelementalHealth.pdf. Accessed July 19, 2010.

Index

Note: Page numbers of article titles are in **boldface** type.

Otolaryngol Clin N Am 44 (2011) 1385–1390
doi:10.1016/S0030-6665(11)00197-6
0030-6665/11/$ – see front matter © 2011 Elsevier Inc. All rights reserved.

oto.theclinics.com

Printed and bound by CPI Group (UK) Ltd, Croydon, CR0 4YY

03/10/2024

01040453-0013

Moving?

Make sure your subscription moves with you!

To notify us of your new address, find your **Clinics Account Number** (located on your mailing label above your name), and contact customer service at:

Email: journalscustomerservice-usa@elsevier.com

800-654-2452 (subscribers in the U.S. & Canada)
314-447-8871 (subscribers outside of the U.S. & Canada)

Fax number: 314-447-8029

Elsevier Health Sciences Division
Subscription Customer Service
3251 Riverport Lane
Maryland Heights, MO 63043

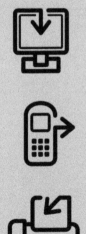

*To ensure uninterrupted delivery of your subscription, please notify us at least 4 weeks in advance of move.

ELSEVIER